Pharmacy in Public Health

Pharmacy in Public Health

Edited by
Janet Krska

School of Pharmacy and Biomolecular Sciences
Liverpool John Moores University
Liverpool
UK

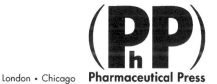

London • Chicago   **Pharmaceutical Press**

Published by Pharmaceutical Press

1 Lambeth High Street, London SE1 7JN, UK
1559 St. Paul Avenue, Gurnee, IL 60031, USA

© Pharmaceutical Press 2011

(PₕP) is a trade mark of Pharmaceutical Press

Pharmaceutical Press is the publishing division of the
Royal Pharmaceutical Society

First published 2011

Typeset by Thomson Digital, Noida, India
Printed in Great Britain by TJ International, Padstow, Cornwall

ISBN 978 0 85369 879 1

A catalogue record for this book is available from the British Library.

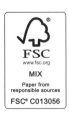

Dedication

For my parents

Contents

Foreword

The vital role that pharmacists play in the provision of healthcare services is widely recognised. This contribution is too often focused simply on the individual patient encounter. In this book, Professor Krska and her co-authors for the first time recognise the importance of pharmacy practice in population health. Public health incorporates many facets, including determining demographic data, estimating the burden of disease, and disease surveillance as well as interventions to improve the health of the population, such as screening and health education. All these are addressed in *Pharmacy in Public Health* by experts in public health, primary care, economics and pharmacy from the United Kingdom and abroad.

Working as they do across primary and secondary care, pharmacists are ideally positioned to play a part in all aspects of public health. This book clearly sets out the pharmacist's role in all aspects of public health. Importantly, it does not confine itself to the United Kingdom but also gives a vital international perspective to the issues.

I hope that, as the first book of its kind, the publication of *Pharmacy in Public Health* will mark the beginning of a new era in pharmaceutical education and practice, where public health and the pharmacist's role is understood and embraced.

Sir Liam Donaldson
Chief Medical Officer (1998–2010)

Preface

I had the idea that a book designed to support pharmacists in developing their public health skills could be useful long before it began to become a reality. The need for it became progressively apparent as more and more elements of public health were taught in undergraduate pharmacy courses, increasing numbers of services aimed at improving public health became established, and ever more pressure to ensure rational, cost-effective and equitable use of medicines was placed upon pharmacists in all sectors of employment.

My own experience began many years ago with involvement in this latter aspect of public health, as a formulary pharmacist. I worked on this with Professor Jim Petrie, who, having led pioneering work in this area, then founded the Scottish Intercollegiate Guideline Network (SIGN), an organisation respected throughout the world. My introduction to evidence-based medicine was certainly at the feet of a master. Much has changed in the way pharmacists practice since those early days, but the principles of rational, cost-effective use of medicines have not. Yet many pharmacists who are involved in developing and implementing formularies and guidelines may not consider these as public health initiatives. This book strives to illustrate that the vast majority of what pharmacists do is public health. It is so much more than just health promotion, as is often thought.

I have been fortunate to have the opportunity to work in a number of different countries, on behalf of the World Health Organization and other health organisations, often in relation to rational prescribing. Whenever I am working in countries around the world, I find there is some good practice from which we in the UK can learn. Although many consider public health pharmacy practice in the UK to be further advanced than most countries, there is always something that we can learn from elsewhere. Therefore this book, while centred on the UK, also deliberately has an international flavour.

As this book goes to print (mid-2010), there has just been a change of government in the UK. Already we hear of potential changes to the organisation of the NHS in England and to local government. Therefore some details, correct at the time of writing, may be inaccurate as you read the book. Conscious of the inevitability of change in organisations that have an impact on public health, I have endeavoured to ensure that this book also emphasises the principles on which public health practice is based, which are not subject to the vagaries of government. What is already established, however, in the latest instructions from the new government, is that the need to enhance quality, innovation, productivity and prevention (QIPP) within the NHS is not going away. Nor is joint working between health and social care – indeed it is of increasing importance – as is strengthening patient and public engagement. Ensuring the clarity of the evidence base for service re-design and development and a specific focus on strengthening the delivery of public health services are mentioned. This book covers much of what we know about public health services involving pharmacy to date and will hopefully provide a useful introduction to these areas.

Editing this book has been a mammoth task for me, but I have learned a great deal along the way. I am grateful to all the authors for their contributions and the staff at Pharmaceutical Press both for commissioning the work and supporting me though the editorial process. My hope is that this book will prove useful to many pharmacists already practising and to undergraduate pharmacy students. My ambition is that it will support and encourage you to contribute to public health, wherever you work.

Janet Krska
September 2010

Acknowledgements

I would like to thank the following staff at Sefton PCT for their kind help in commenting on a number of chapters in this book during its development: Linda Turner, Consultant in Public Health; Katie Dutton, Partnership Development Manager; Brendan Prescott, Lead Adviser in Pharmaceutical Primary Care, and also Paul Spivey, Consultant Pharmacist, World Health Organization who reviewed several chapters. I am also grateful to The School of Pharmacy and Life Sciences, The Robert Gordon University, for permission to use teaching materials in Chapter 9.

About the editor

Janet Krska is currently Professor of Pharmacy Practice at Liverpool John Moores University and Honorary Adviser in Public Health at NHS Sefton Primary Care Trust. She has experience of all sectors of pharmacy and has published widely on many topics relevant to public health. Previous posts include formulary management pharmacist (Grampian Health Board), Consultant in Pharmaceutical Public Health (Grampian Health Board) and Public Health Development Pharmacist (Angus LHCC, NHS Tayside).

List of contributors

Claire Anderson BPharm PhD MCPP FRPharmS
Professor of Social Pharmacy, Division of Social Research in Medicines and Health, School of Pharmacy, University of Nottingham, UK

Carol Armour BPharm(Hons) PhD FPS
Associate Dean (Research Career Development) Faculty of Medicine and Professor, Faculty of Pharmacy, University of Sydney, New South Wales, Australia

Janet Atherton MB BS MSc FFPH
Director of Public Health for NHS Sefton and Sefton Council, UK

John Bell AM BPharm FPS FRPharmS FACPP MSHP
Vice-President International Pharmaceutical Federation and Principal Advisor – Self Care Program, Pharmaceutical Society of Australia, Deakin, Australia

Alison Blenkinsopp BPharm PhD FRPharmS OBE
School of Pharmacy, Professor of Pharmacy Practice, Keele University, UK

Christine M Bond BPharm MEd PhD FRPharmS FFPH FHEA
Head of Centre of Academic Primary Care, University of Aberdeen, UK

Brian Godman BSc
Research Fellow, Institute for Pharmacological Research, 'Mario Negri', Milano, Italy, and Division of Clinical Pharmacology, Karolinska Institutet, Karolinska University Hospital, Stockholm, Sweden

Fiona Harris LLM MSc (Public Health) BPharm MRPharmS FFPH
Joint Consultant in Public Health (Sutton), NHS Sutton and Merton and the London Borough of Sutton, UK

Dyfrig A Hughes BPharm MSc PhD MRPharmS
Professor in Pharmacoeconomics, Centre for Economics and Policy in Health, Bangor University, UK

Peter Knapp RGN PhD
Senior Lecturer, School of Healthcare, University of Leeds, UK

Ines Krass BPharm Dip Hosp Pharm Grad Dip Educ Studies PhD
Head of Pharmacy Practice, The University of Sydney, Australia

Adam J Mackridge PhD MRPharmS PGCert FHEA
Senior Lecturer in Pharmacy Practice, School of Pharmacy and Biomolecular Sciences, Liverpool John Moores University, UK

Charles Morecroft PhD PGCert FHEA FRPharmS
Principal Lecturer in Pharmacy Practice, School of Pharmacy and Biomolecular Sciences, Liverpool John Moores University, UK

Penelope A Phillips-Howard SRN PhD FRSPH
Reader in Public Health Centre for Public Health, Liverpool John Moores University, Liverpool, UK

David Pfleger BSc MPH MRPharmS
Senior Lecturer in Pharmaceutical Public Health and Consultant in Pharmaceutical Public Health, NHS Grampian, School of Pharmacy and Life Sciences, Robert Gordon University, Aberdeen UK

Roger Walker BPharm PhD FRPharmS FFPH
Professor of Pharmacy Practice, Welsh School of Pharmacy, Cardiff University and Consultant in Pharmaceutical Public Health, Public Health Wales, Temple of Peace and Health, Cardiff, UK

Margaret C Watson MSc Epidemiol MSc Clin Pharm PhD
Senior Research Fellow, Centre of Academic Primary Care, University of Aberdeen, UK

Abbreviations

ACMD	Advisory Council on the Misuse of Drugs
ADQ	average daily quantity
ADR	adverse drug reaction
AIDS	auto-immune deficiency syndrome
APC	area prescribing committee
APHO	Association of Public Health Observatories
ARR	absolute risk reduction
BMI	body mass index
BP	blood pressure
CEA	cost-effectiveness analysis
CHD	coronary heart disease
CMA	cost-minimisation analysis
CUA	cost-utility analysis
CVD	cardiovascular disease
DALY	disability-adjusted life-year
DDD	defined daily dose
DOE	disease-oriented evidence
DoH	Department of Health
DOTS	directly observed treatment, short-course
DPH	Director of Public Health
DTC	drug and therapeutics committee
DXA	dual-energy X-ray absorptiometry
EBM	evidence-based medicine
EHC	emergency hormonal contraception
EMA	European Medicines Agency
EU	European Union
FOBT	faecal occult blood test
GHS	General Household Survey
GP	general practitioner
GPRD	General Practice Research Database
GSL	general sales list
H_2RA	histamine H_2-receptor antagonists

HDA	Health Development Agency
HDL	high density lipoprotein
HES	Hospital Episode Statistics
HIA	health equity impact assessement
HIV	human immunodeficiency virus
HNA	health needs assessment
HPA	Health Protection Agency
HPV	human papillomavirus
HRQOL	health-related quality of life
HSE	Health Survey for England
HTA	health technology assessment
IMD	index of multiple deprivation
IPSF	International Pharmaceutical Students' Federation
JSNA	joint strategic needs assessment
LDL	low density lipoprotein
LWI	Live Well Initiative
MFC	malaria fact card
MHRA	Medicines and Healthcare products Regulatory Agency
MMR	measles, mumps, rubella
MRSA	methicillin-resistant *Staphylococcus aureus*
NHS	National Health Service
NICE	National Institute for Health and Clinical Excellence
NLRS	National Laboratory Reporting Scheme
NNH	number needed to harm
NNT	number needed to treat
NPSA	National Patient Safety Agency
(NS-SeC)	National Statistics Socioeconomic Classification
NRT	nicotine replacement therapy
NSAID	non-steroidal anti-inflammatory drug
NSP	needle and syringe programme
NTG	national treatment guideline
OA	output area
OECD	Organisation for Economic Co-operation and Development
ONS	Office of National Statistics
OR	odds ratio
OTC	over-the-counter
PCT	Primary Care Trust
PGD	patient group direction
PIED	performance and image enhancing drug
POC	point of care
POEM	patient-oriented evidence that matters
POM	prescription-only medicine
POPP	Partnerships for Older People Projects

PPI	proton pump inhibitor
PPV	positive predictive value
PROM	patient-related outcome measure
PSA	prostate-specific antigen
PYLL	potential years life lost
QALY	quality-adjusted life-year
QOF	quality and outcomes framework
RCT	randomised controlled trial
ROC	receiver operating characteristic
RPSGB	Royal Pharmaceutical Society of Great Britain
RR	relative risk
RRR	relative risk reduction
SIGN	Scottish Intercollegiate Guidelines Network
SMC	Scottish Medicines Consortium
SMR	standard mortality ratio
SOA	super output area
SOP	standard operating procedure
SSRI	selective serotonin reuptake inhibitor
STI	sexually transmitted infection
TB	tuberculosis
TC	total cholesterol
TIA	transient ischaemic attack
UKPHR	United Kingdom Public Health Register
VSO	Voluntary Service Overseas
WHO	World Health Organization
YCS	Yellow Card Scheme

SECTION 1

Overview of public health

1

Public health in the UK

Janet Krska and Janet Atherton

What is public health?

There are many definitions of public health, but all have a similar basis. The one currently widely used in the UK is: 'The science and art of preventing disease, prolonging life and promoting health through the organised efforts and informed choices of society, organisations, public and private, communities and individuals.'[1] This was first developed in the 1920s, but still describes what public health involves, not just in the UK, but worldwide.

Health, as defined by the World Health Organization (WHO) is: 'a sense of physical, mental and social well-being and not just the absence of disease or infirmity.' Health is a continuum, from complete wellness to chronic, disabling illness and is experienced differently by everyone. Someone with a chronic illness can still describe themselves as feeling 'well'.

The term 'public' refers to individual members of the community, social groups in which individuals play a part, and organisations both local and national, including government. The organised efforts of these groups thus include a wide spectrum of activities that influence global and national policies, such as reducing carbon emissions, creating fairer societies and include legislative measures, for example, banning smoking in public places, educational programmes and commissioning and providing social services. Many organisations also help and support individuals to make informed choices associated with improved health, for example, minimising risky behaviour or supporting healthy lifestyles. They also aim to ensure equity and equality of opportunities.

What does public health involve?

Public health activities are often divided into three main areas: health protection and prevention, health and social care, and health improvement (Box 1.1). Much of what public health seeks to do can thus be described as:

- assessing the health of a population through information gathering
- implementing measures designed to protect the public from harm and to prevent ill health
- identifying evidence to support a range of approaches to improve population health
- ensuring equitable provision of efficient and effective services designed to achieve good health
- monitoring the impact of interventions, services and policies on the population's health.

Box 1.1 *Domains of public health*

Health protection and prevention	Health and social care	Health improvement
Disease and injury prevention	Quality	Employment
Communicable disease control	Clinical effectiveness	Housing
Environmental health hazards	Efficiency	Family/community
Emergency planning	Service planning	Education
Audit and evaluation	Inequalities/exclusion	
Clinical governance	Lifestyles	

Reproduced with permission from the Faculty of Public Health.

Public health initiatives must therefore be based on information about the health of populations, including local patterns of disease (see Chapter 4), causes of mortality and morbidity, existing infrastructure and priorities. All these differ both between areas within a country, e.g. the four home countries of UK, more locally e.g. between Primary Care Trusts (PCTs) and also between countries. Varying disease patterns are affected by differences in the underlying determinants of health (see Chapter 2). These differences, together with differences in healthcare provision dictate differing needs of populations and therefore different approaches to public health services (see Chapter 5).

Public health policy and structure in the UK

Until 1974, local government authorities were responsible for the health of local communities, through medical officers of health. This responsibility then moved to local health authorities, but the foundations of current public health practice were not laid down until 1988 by the policy paper *Public Health in England*. This followed two major outbreaks of infectious diseases in hospitals, which identified that there was a lack of accountability and capacity to respond to such incidents. Therefore two important roles were created which are still key to ensuring the health of local communities: the local Director of Public Health (see page 11) and Consultant in Communicable Disease Control (see page 11). At this time the director was based in the district health authority, which was hospital based but National Health Service (NHS) reforms in 2001 resulted in these posts moving closer to primary care, where they could more effectively work to improve the health of local communities. Currently many directors have joint appointments between local government and local health organisations; thus the role has evolved from government-centred, through health-centred to a combination of both. The current position more closely reflects the elements of public health illustrated in Box 1.1, which span both government and health organisations although the position may revert to local government in future.

At a national level, policy that affects population health is developed by government, through health ministers and civil servants, working at a Department of Health (DoH) or equivalent ministry. The latter includes Chief Medical, Nursing and Pharmaceutical Officers. The Secretary of State for health or equivalent has responsibility to ensure adequate provision of health services for their country's population, although this is devolved to chief executives within NHS organisations. The public health directors support the chief executives in fulfilling these obligations.

Health inequalities

Health inequalities were first identified when information started to be collected about causes of death and occupations in the 1830s. However, health inequalities are not a phenomenon of history, they are still with us today. In 1980 the *Report of the Working Group on Inequalities in Health* (also known as the Black report after its chairman Sir Douglas Black) was published, which demonstrated the extent to which ill health and death were unequally distributed among the population of Britain.[2] The report concluded that these inequalities are mainly attributable to social inequalities influencing health: income, education, housing, diet, employment and conditions of work, which are now reflected in our understanding of the determinants of health (see Chapter 2). Many of the Black report's

37 recommendations have been taken up by subsequent governments. For example, Black recommended the extension of non-smoking areas in public places and wide availability of smoking cessation advice.

At the time, the issues raised by the Black report were never addressed and health inequalities continued to increase. The *Health of the Nation* strategy, implemented in 1992, did provide for the first time a strategic attempt to improve the overall health of the population. Unfortunately the strategy failed to tackle the underlying determinants of health and in 1998, an *Independent Inquiry into Inequalities in Health*, chaired by Sir Donald Acheson, Chief Medical Officer, was published.[3] The Acheson report further demonstrated the differences in health outcomes between social classes and was a major influence on the 1999 White Paper *Saving Lives: Our healthier nation*.[4] This document aimed to tackle poor health by 'improving the health of everyone, and of the worst off in particular'. It required people, communities and government to work together in partnership to improve health, stated that 'individuals and their families need to be properly informed about risk to make decisions', and required local authorities to work in partnership with the NHS. Partnership working (Chapter 8) is now seen as vital to improving public health. *Saving Lives: Our Healthier Nation* also resulted in the establishment of the Health Development Agency (HDA), a statutory body charged with raising the standards and quality of public health provision. The work of the HDA, which sought to develop the evidence base to improve health and reduce inequalities, has since been subsumed into the National Institute for Health and Clinical Excellence (NICE; see page 10).

More recently, a further report (*Securing Our Future Health: Taking a long term view*) was commissioned in 2002 from Sir Derek Wanless, a statistician, to assess the resources required for the NHS to achieve these aims.[5] This report argued that the NHS was providing a national sickness service and outlined three different costing models, depending on to what extent the general public engaged with the need to improve their own health. Wanless argued that changing public behaviour involves changing social norms and that this may involve legislation. His follow-up report in 2004 (*Securing Good Health for the Whole Population: Final report*) set out the challenges that the government would face for the public to become 'fully engaged' with improving their own health.[1] Smoking, obesity and health inequalities were identified as major threats to improving the population's health. Wanless advocated ensuring access to personalised high quality information advice and support to help individuals decide whether to engage and stated that health services must 'evolve from dealing with acute problems through more effective control of chronic conditions to promoting the maintenance of good health.'

The subsequent White Paper: *Choosing Health: Making health choices easier*, published in 2004[6] had three core principles: enabling people to make informed choices, supporting people to make healthier choices and effective working partnerships between government, health and other organisations. It set out six priorities for action:

- reduce the numbers of people who smoke
- reduce obesity and improve diet and nutrition
- increase exercise
- encourage and support sensible drinking
- improve sexual health
- improve mental health.

Key targets, for example, reducing inequalities by 10%, as measured by life expectancy at birth and infant mortality, were set.[7] In 2004, specific geographical areas on which efforts should be focused were identified, termed 'spearhead populations', which had the worst health and deprivation indicators in England. The conditions leading to differences in life expectancy between spearheads and other populations were identified as cardiovascular disease, cancer and respiratory disease. Interventions designed to reduce this difference which are targeted towards these populations are smoking cessation, control of blood pressure, cholesterol, blood sugar and anticoagulant therapy in patients with atrial fibrillation.

However, the Marmot review: *Fair Society, Healthy Lives* published in 2010[8] showed that, despite continued efforts to reduce health inequalities, these remain and continue to differ between regions of England. Social inequalities underpin the determinants of health, thus lead to health inequalities (see Chapter 2). This review identified the most effective, evidence-based strategies for reducing health inequalities in England and recommended wide-ranging, universal action, of a scale and intensity in proportion to the level of disadvantage. Marmot's recommendations extend from early years education through access to life-long learning, good jobs with minimum income, improving communities and prioritising investment in ill health prevention and health promotion. To achieve this latter goal, involving stakeholders, partnership working and local service design and delivery are recommended (see Chapters 6, 8 and 9).

Marmot advocates that all interventions should have an evidence-based evaluation framework and a health equity impact assessment (HIA). This involves assessing the potential impact of a policy taking account of the direct and wider determinants of health on the health of the whole population served, as well as sub-groups within it. The purpose of a HIA is to ensure that a given policy does not further widen health inequalities.

Importantly, recently the focus of public health has shifted more towards overall health and well-being, encompassing an overall approach to living within our communities.

Three further independent reports illustrate how behaviour change could be tackled,[9] discuss the role of government in improving health and well-being[10] and make recommendations about how to deliver health and well-being.[11]

Effect of devolution

Devolution in 1998 meant that separate government of the health service by the four individual home countries making up the UK required different policies, which could be based on different needs and approaches. In Scotland, the White Paper *Partnership for Care*, published in 2003,[12] highlighted the death rates in Scotland from cancer and coronary heart disease, which were among the highest in the world, but also recognised community pharmacy as having a central role in improving health. As in England, empowerment of the people and partnership working were key measures. A new organisation was also established in 2003, NHS Health Scotland, to provide leadership and joint working to improve health and reduce health inequalities in Scotland.

After devolution, a strategy was developed in Wales, based on the publication *Better Health, Better Wales* (1998), to improve health and reduce inequalities.[13] Like Scotland, Wales too established a national organisation for public health in 2003, the National Public Health Service for Wales. This is part of a new trust, Public Health Wales, which provides resources information and advice to the Welsh Assembly government, local health boards and local authorities. In Northern Ireland, public health is the responsibility of the Chief Medical Officer for the Department of Health, Social Services and Public Safety. In addition, an Institute of Public Health promotes cooperation for public health between Northern Ireland and the Republic of Ireland.

Public health practice in the UK

In their everyday practice, all healthcare professionals, including pharmacists, are familiar with assessing the needs of individuals, drawing on evidence to provide services to meet those needs in a cost-effective way and monitoring the outcomes of the interventions they have made. Some of these interventions are preventive, such as advising someone to stop smoking or prescribing aspirin to a patient after a myocardial infarction. Public health uses the same general principles of assessing need, drawing on evidence and monitoring outcomes, but in populations, rather than in individuals. Interventions may be designed and developed locally, or nationally, but to be effective must still be delivered or implemented in individuals. Therefore there is a need for public health expertise at all levels of society and healthcare practice (see below).

Public health activities require the amassing of information, in order to assess the need for interventions and their impact and to respond to public health problems within the community. This requires the collection of data or 'intelligence' about lifestyle, disease and also vital events – births, deaths and stillbirths. 'Intelligence gathering' is an important public health role (see Chapter 4).

To achieve improvements in health, public health activities and services must address the root causes of illness and disease, including the social, environmental, biological and psychological factors that impact on health and well-being (see Chapter 2). Therefore joint working (see Chapter 8) and involving the people actually affected by an issue or problem, or their representatives, are important elements of public health work. While involving the public increases the effectiveness of interventions, public health directors and practitioners must also act as advocates for their population (see Chapter 8). They must ensure equitable distribution of services. Equitable distribution is based on need, not demand and is not the same as equal distribution. Equal distribution of resources could result in those with greatest need having insufficient, while those with the least need have excess. Inequitable distribution is unjust, unfair and may be unequal, but is also remediable. Much of public health practice focuses on ensuring equity. Given that equity is based on need, assessing the needs of populations is also a major part of public health practice (see Chapter 6).

Public health working at different levels

Three levels of public health working have been identified: specialist, practitioner and wider workforce. Specialists include those with higher qualifications in public health, working in positions that are mainly focused on the health of populations. Specialists work strategically at international, national, regional and local levels. Practitioners provide health interventions for individuals that ultimately affect the population's health, while the wider workforce includes a huge variety of individuals who may affect health through their work but are not regarded as health professionals. These include people involved in education, journalism and policy making as well as healthcare.

International level

The World Health Organization (WHO) was established in 1948 and is the public health arm of the United Nations. It is responsible for providing leadership on global health matters, shaping the health research agenda, setting norms and standards, articulating evidence-based policy options, providing technical support to countries and monitoring and assessing health trends. A wide variety of other international agencies, e.g. the World Bank, UNICEF, government aid departments (such as the UK Department for International Development), the European Community, Australian AID, USAID and non-government organisations such as WaterAid and Medicins sans Frontières also support public health development internationally.

National level

Each of the home countries of the UK has a department of health or similar organisation which has responsibility for health protection, health improvement and health inequalities. This includes issues such as pandemic influenza, seasonal influenza, patient safety, tobacco, obesity, drugs, sexual health and international health. In England the DoH develop policies to improve the prevention and control of infectious diseases and other environmental threats to the health of the population. However, the DoH is supported by the work of the Health Protection Agency (HPA), which maintains surveillance and provides information and advice to organisations and individuals. It covers health hazards and emergencies caused by infectious diseases, hazardous chemicals, poisons and radiation (see Chapter 12). All four home countries and the Republic of Ireland are also supported by a network of 12 public health observatories. The observatories gather and analyse information on people's health, lifestyle and use of healthcare, which is available to health organisations and the public. These data are used for a variety of purposes including:

- monitoring health and disease trends and highlighting areas for action
- identifying gaps in health information
- assessing the impact of health inequalities
- evaluating progress in improving health and reducing inequality
- looking ahead to give early warning of public health problems.

Another important body that influences public health practice in England is NICE. NICE provide guidelines on public health initiatives, which are assessed by a public health intervention advisory committee. An example guidance document is *Brief Interventions and Referral for Smoking Cessation in Primary Care and Other Settings*.[14] Guidance such as this is developed by reviewing published evidence derived from epidemiological studies and assessing its quality to make recommendations (see Chapters 4 and 7). NICE also provides clinical guidance, on a wide range of medical conditions but, importantly for public health, it also publishes health technology appraisals. These appraise the evidence for a particular intervention, to ensure equitable availability of the intervention and cost-effective use of resources.

Setting standards of public health practice is done at a UK level by the Faculty of Public Health and other bodies (see Chapter 3).

Regional level

There may be public health organisations that cover parts of a country, such as exist in regions of England. At this level in England, regional public health directors currently are joint posts between the health authority and government, and who lead teams of people with a wide range of expertise in diverse fields. These may include public health medicine, nursing, health visiting, dentistry, pharmacy, social science, statistics, environmental health and health promotion. The functions of the public health departments of the regions in England are:

- the development of a cross-government and cross-sector approach to tackling the wider determinants of health
- informing regional work on economic regeneration, education, employment and transport
- ensuring there is a proper health contribution to local strategic partnerships
- accountability for the protection of health (including against communicable diseases and environmental hazards) across the region
- making sure the public health function is properly managed at local level
- emergency and disaster planning and management.

There is a statutory requirement to have a mechanism of monitoring and dealing with communicable disease at regional level, delegated to a designated medical officer, the Consultant in Communicable Disease Control. This role requires liaison with other agencies outside the NHS, such as local authorities, veterinary, agriculture, water and the food service industry. The consultant is also responsible for ensuring that records of certain infectious diseases are collected through the disease notification system. These are sent to national centres for collation in the UK. It is also the public health department's responsibility to distribute information about known health hazards to the public.

Local level

At a more local level, smaller healthcare organisations such as PCTs in England also employ a Director of Public Health, and again many posts are joint with local government. There is no requirement for this person to be medically qualified, but they must be registered as a public health specialist (see Chapter 3). The director publishes an annual report independent of their organisation, which gives information about the health of the local community. It contains reliable epidemiological information about the local population, such as prevalence of diseases, lifestyles, access to services, social and economic factors that influence health locally and it illustrates any health inequalities. The information is gathered by local public health intelligence departments, drawing on the work of the regional observatory, together with other specially collected data. This report facilitates the development and implementation of local plans and strategies by local agencies working together, to tackle locally important issues and priorities.

Health promotion as a discipline is very closely linked with public health and public health departments also employ specialists in health promotion to advise on campaigns, including social marketing (see Chapter 4). Pharmacists as specialists in medicines management are often located within public health departments, because not only are medicines a health resource that needs to be managed ethically and cost-effectively but also because community pharmacy has such an important opportunistic role to play in promoting and protecting health. One important aspect of medicines distribution dealt with at local level is the cascade of information about product recalls.

Local public health departments need to work with a wide range of organisations to deliver improvements in health. These include: social services, local authorities, voluntary sector, police, care homes, schools and other education institutions and transport organisations. For example, local government organisations employ environmental health officers whose job includes the development, coordination and implementation of public health policies to ensure that the health of the public is protected. Their remit covers food safety and nutrition, housing conditions, environment and workplace health and safety.

Operational level: public health practitioners and the wider workforce

Every healthcare professional who comes into contact with the public has a public health function. Health visitors play a major role in promoting healthy prenatal and postnatal lifestyles, providing immunisation to children and many other activities, such as smoking cessation or weight management clinics. Primary care medical practitioners organise clinics within their practices which enable chronic diseases to be managed, including screening for associated problems. Practice nurses run well-person clinics, provide immunisation to those at risk of influenza and take cervical smears for screening against cervical cancer. Dietitians provide advice on healthy eating. Community pharmacists provide harm minimisation services to drug misusers, smoking cessation advice, advice on reducing risks from medicines and much more. The wider workforce includes a variety of staff, such as teachers, local government officers and social care staff, often working in partnership with health organisations.

It is important to remember that although the focus of public health work is mainly in the community, hospital workers also have a vital role to play. Infection control policies and medicines management policies are crucial in hospital. Secondary care staff are involved in providing screening programmes. Giving smoking cessation advice and support can be extremely effective in hospital, where there is a 'no smoking' policy, particularly in patients whose admission was due to a smoking-related disease. Hospitals also collect important data used for public health practice and evaluate the impact of novel ways of working.

Working together to improve public health

All the levels of practice are needed if the overall health of the world's population is to improve, since public health involves global, national and local policies and practices, as well as the delivery of services and interventions to individuals. Multi-agency working is also important because improved public health and well-being will not be achieved by healthcare organisations working in isolation. Box 1.2 illustrates the necessity of

---

Box 1.2 *How public health works: tuberculosis management*

Tuberculosis (TB) has been increasing in prevalence in the UK since the mid-1990s, with 8497 cases reported in 2006. TB can be fatal (about 250 people die each year from TB in England), is difficult to treat and is not controlled by BCG vaccination programmes. A national action plan launched in England in 2004 aimed to increase awareness of the problem, monitor trends in cases, provide high quality laboratory facilities for diagnosis and ensure consistent management, including supervised consumption of drug therapy to ensure compliance, if needed. The plan also includes screening of high risk individuals and contacts of infected persons, as well as international collaboration to minimise the spread to and from other countries. The development of drug resistance required national guidelines on selection of therapy. Furthermore, because the rise in TB is associated with HIV, a national HIV-testing policy for patients with TB was also established.

Treating individuals without the additional public health measures would reduce the overall effectiveness and vice versa. Public health supports other healthcare practice and healthcare practice supports public health.

different levels of practice, while Box 1.3 illustrates, through a strategy designed to reduce smoking, the importance of multiple agencies and activities in achieving improved health. Many public health organisations and individual practitioners were involved in lobbying for and influencing government policy on smoking in UK countries and the smoking ban in public places can be regarded as a major public health achievement, which should contribute to the continuing decline in smoking.

Box 1.3 *Public health in a wider context: tobacco control strategy*[15]

The government in England has devised a strategy that aims to stop young people starting to smoke, help smokers to quit and protect people from tobacco-related harm. It sets targets for each of these objectives and outlines methods for achieving these, which include initiatives in legislation and education, as well as service provision.

Legislative changes will include:

- making tobacco less affordable
- removing tobacco from display in shops, prohibiting vending machines and greater enforcement of regulations about sale
- extending controls on advertising
- extending smoke-free areas.

Educational initiatives will include:

- improved labelling of tobacco products
- developing school-based initiatives
- promoting smoke-free communities.

Services provided will include:

- offering and promoting more opportunities for quitters
- ensuring pharmacological therapies are widely available and promoted appropriately
- targeting smoking during pregnancy for special support.

Coordination of public health responses to emergencies

Another example of how organisations work together at different levels is the public health response to emergencies, which is a health protection function. Emergency situations come in a wide variety of guises; for example, local flooding, major accidents or outbreaks of infections. Public health staff must contribute to emergency planning for such incidents. Emergency planning requires coordination of public health practice at all levels and between many organisations. At a global level the United Nations, governments and non-government organisations may provide aid immediately and longer term after an international incident but require coordination. This is achieved through the WHO which has the mandate and a department to coordinate the health response in a health emergency or natural disaster.

In the UK, the NHS provides emergency planning guidance. Strategic command arrangements are also needed to ensure 'command, control and coordination' exists between different healthcare services in primary and secondary care. This ensures a structured and cohesive response to the emergency. Three levels of planning are recognised – strategic, tactical and operational, also known as Gold, Silver and Bronze. Gold or strategic leaders have overall command of resources and must monitor response to an emergency incident. Tactical decisions are taken by Silver managers, who also plan and coordinate tasks. Operational (Bronze) leaders implement the plan and control the resources required within their local area.

Emergency planning must also consider business continuity planning, to ensure that there is a seamless recovery from a major disruption. Emergency planning may require additional training, co-opting of personnel to deal with either emergency or ongoing situations, perhaps performing tasks normally not within their role. An example of this occurred during the swine flu epidemic in 2009, when public health staff at all levels were either involved in planning the response or in delivering it. Pharmacists also had input at all levels down to supply of antiviral medicines without prescription or providing vaccinations. During emergencies, such as this, both public health intelligence and regular planning are vital. Hence Gold, Silver and Bronze planning meetings were held daily, weekly or less frequently, depending on level of alert, at various levels throughout the whole NHS, using information obtained through a variety of sources (see Chapter 4).

A key feature of emergencies is the need for communicating information, both from high levels to those working on the front line and vice versa. For example, during the swine flu epidemic pharmacists needed to receive information on implementing the strategy and also provide information on the number of antivirals issued on a daily basis.

In addition, public health directors are responsible for providing scientific and technical advice to a multi-agency strategic coordination centre, often leading a science and technical advice cell (STAC). The cell provides advice to the Gold leader in case of emergencies.

Skills required for public health practice

In some countries, public health is a separate health profession, taught at undergraduate level, whereas public health in the UK developed historically as a speciality within the medical profession. Given the diversity of public health practice, however, there is a need for skills development among a range of disciplines and at a range of levels. A public health skills and career framework has been developed,[16] which sets out competences and underpinning knowledge for different career levels in four core areas and five specialist areas (Tables 1.1 and 1.2). Pharmacy fits into this, along with other health disciplines, depending on the level at which individuals practice (see Chapter 3).

Table 1.1 Career levels for public health practitioners: framework levels		
Level	**Summarised role**	**Examples of staff working at this level**
1	Provides specific public health activities under direction	Volunteer workers
2	Provides range of defined public health activities under guidance	Healthcare assistant, community pharmacy support staff
3	As 2, but may assist in training, have responsibility for resources, set priorities or make decisions	Stop smoking adviser, health promotion assistant, senior community pharmacy support staff
4	Has responsibility for specific area(s) of public health with guidance	Health visitor assistant, teacher
5	Has responsibility for specific area(s) of public health, contributes to multi-agency working	Smoking cessation coordinator, registered nurse, community pharmacist
6	Has autonomy and responsibility in coordinating complex work in area(s) of public health	Specialist in community health nursing, senior health improvement officer, pharmacy public health facilitator
7	Leads on areas of public health work	Specialist smoking adviser, health visitor, pharmacy public health specialist
8	High level of expertise in specific area of work, or broad programmes, sets strategic direction in own area of work	Deputy director of public health, head of information in public health organisation, nurse consultant, lead pharmacy public health specialist
9	Sets strategic direction across organisations, provides multi-sectoral leadership	Director of public health, director of public health organisation

Adapted from the public health skills and career framework.[16]

Table 1.2 Areas of competence for public health practitioners	
Core areas	**Non-core (defined) areas**
Surveillance and assessment of the population's health and well-being	Health improvement
Assessing the evidence of effectiveness of interventions, programmes and services to improve population health and well-being	Health protection
Policy and strategy development and implementation for population health and well-being	Public health intelligence
Leadership and collaborative working for population health and well-being	Academic public health
	Health and social care quality
Adapted from the public health skills and career framework.[16]	

References

1. Wanless D. *Securing Good Health for the Whole Population: Final report.* London: HMSO, 2004. http://www.dh.gov.uk/en/Publicationsandstatistics/Publications/PublicationsPolicyAndGuidance/DH_4074426.
2. Black D. *Inequalities in Health: Report of a research working group.* London: Department of Health and Social Services, 1980. http://www.sochealth.co.uk/Black/black.htm.
3. Acheson D. *Independent Inquiry into Inequalities in Health Report.* London: The Stationery Office, 1998. http://www.archive.official-documents.co.uk/document/doh/ih/contents.htm.
4. Department of Health. *Saving Lives: Our healthier nation.* London: Department of Health, 1999. http://www.dh.gov.uk/en/Publicationsandstatistics/Publications/PublicationsPolicyAndGuidance/DH_4118614.
5. Wanless D. *Securing Our Future Health: Taking a long-term view. Final report.* London: HM Treasury, 2002. http://www.hm-treasury.gov.uk/wanless.
6. Department of Health. *Choosing Health: Making healthy choices easier.* London: Department of Health, 2004. http://www.dh.gov.uk/en/Publicationsandstatistics/Publications/PublicationsPolicyAndGuidance/DH_4094550.
7. Department of Health. *Tackling Health Inequalities: A programme for action.* London: Department of Health, 2004.
8. The Marmot Review. *Fair Society, Healthy Lives.* London: The Marmot Review, 2010. www.ucl.ac.uk/whitehallII/pdf/FairSocietyHealthyLives.pdf
9. Mulgan G. *Influencing Public Behaviour to Improve Health and Well-Being.* London: Department of Health, 2010.http://www.dh.gov.uk/en/Publicationsandstatistics/Publications/PublicationsPolicyAndGuidance/DH_111696.
10. Reeves R. *A Liberal Dose? Health and Well-Being: The role of the state.* London: Department of Health, 2010. http://www.dh.gov.uk/en/Publicationsandstatistics/Publications/PublicationsPolicyAndGuidance/DH_111697.
11. Bernstein H, Cosford P, Willams A. *Enabling Effective Delivery of Health and Well-Being.* London: Department of Health, 2010. http://www.dh.gov.uk/en/Publicationsandstatistics/Publications/PublicationsPolicyAndGuidance/DH_111692.
12. *Partnership for Care: Scotland's health white paper.* Edinburgh: Scottish Executive, 2003. http://www.scotland.gov.uk/Publications/2003/02/16476/18730.

13. *Better Health, Better Wales.* The Stationery Office, 1998. http://www.wales.nhs.uk/publications/stratframe98_e.pdf.
14. National Institute for Health and Clinical Excellence. *Brief Interventions and Referral for Smoking Cessation in Primary Care and Other Settings.* London: NICE, 2006. http://guidance.nice.org.uk/PH1.
15. HM Government. *A Smokefree Future: A comprehensive tobacco control strategy for England.* London: Department of Health, 2010. http://www.dh.gov.uk/en/Publicationsandstatistics/Publications/PublicationsPolicyAndGuidance/DH_111749
16. Skills for Health/Public Health Resource Unit. *Public Health Skills and Career Framework.* London: PHRU, 2008. http://www.phru.nhs.uk/pages/phd/public_health_career_framework.htm

2

Determinants of health

Roger Walker

Background

The 20th century saw significant improvements in health and longevity, with life expectancy in the UK improving in every decade after 1840. A baby boy or girl born in England in 1900 could expect to live for 45 and 49 years of age respectively. By 2009[1] this had increased to in excess of 75 years for males and 80 years for females. Over the same period, infant mortality fell from 140 per 1000 live births in 1900 to under 5. The health of people in all social classes is now better than ever before and has improved consistently. However, there is concern that the gap in health between those who are 'rich' and those who are 'poor' also continues to increase, as does that of those who live in 'rich' and 'poor' areas. This inequality in health is not unique to the UK and occurs in most countries worldwide.

There is now general acceptance that inequalities in health are founded in poverty and material wealth. Investment and improvement in the healthcare service for 'poor' people can play a significant part in reducing these inequalities in health. However, taking steps to reduce differences in material standards of living at work, in the home and in everyday social and community life are of even greater importance.[2] The factors that have the clearest links with this additional burden of ill health are low income, unhealthy behaviour and poor housing and environmental amenities.[3] These and related issues, often referred to as the wider determinants of health, are the focus of this chapter. Once these wider determinants have been discussed, along with other markers of socioeconomic status and health, their utility in measuring and monitoring deprivation will be considered.

The relevance of a knowledge of the wider determinants of health to the health of the individual patient and the work of a practising pharmacist, may initially be unclear. However, the degree of success a pharmacist, or other healthcare worker, may have in improving the health of any given individual will be influenced by the wider determinants of health that impact on the individual. Take the example of two males, both aged 45 years and with poor inhaler technique. The person who lives in poor quality, overcrowded, damp, temporary housing with no job and lacking family/partner support and integration into any social or community network will present a different challenge to the wealthy, well-educated individual wanting to improve his respiratory health but faced with none of the problems described for his counterpart. If the challenges facing the individual from a deprived background are combined with an erratic and hazardous lifestyle that includes smoking and drinking to excess, it is clear that endeavours to improve a questionable inhaler technique pale into insignificance in the wider context of the challenges he faces.

Determinants of health

Health is influenced in a positive or negative way by a variety of factors and a model to describe the many interactions was first conceptualised by Dahlgren and Whitehead (Figure 2.1).[4]

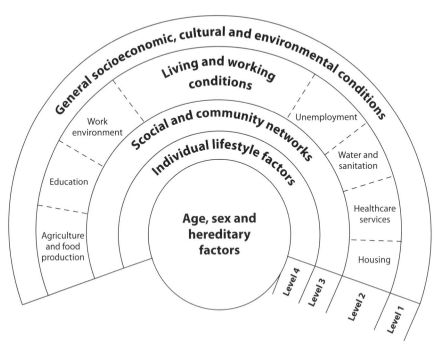

Figure 2.1 Determinants of health, based on the original model of Dahlgren and Whitehead.[4] With permission from Dahlgren G, Whitehead M. *Policies and Strategies to Promote Social Equity in Health*. Stockholm: Institute for Future Studies, 1991.

Their model maps the relationship between the individual, their environment and disease. At the centre of the model is the individual with their age, gender and genetic make-up, i.e. the non-modifiable factors that influence health and disease. Surrounding this central core are a range of modifiable factors. These include personal behaviour and the ways of living (lifestyle) that can promote or damage health. Typical of these factors are smoking, alcohol intake, eating habits, exercise and sexual behaviour. These, in turn, are influenced by social and community factors that determine the norms of a community, the level of crime, social inclusion/exclusion and whether there is support (or not) for the individual at difficult times. Employment, working conditions and the built environment such as housing and safe streets, together with the natural environment and the global ecosystem can all be further incorporated in the model as identifiable factors that impact on health.

The mechanism and interrelationships through which these determinants influence health is not clear. We know they contribute to health inequalities between social groups and can influence health both directly and indirectly. For example, damp housing can contribute directly to respiratory disease, while poor education can limit employment opportunities, increase the likelihood that eventual employment will be poorly paid and thereby put the individual in a poverty trap with its adverse impact on health. Moreover, because poverty is linked to poor housing, poor diet and poor access to healthcare services, there are many potential contributory factors to ill health and the dominant route may vary from individual to individual.

Non-modifiable factors

These are the determinants of health that are at the centre of the model shown in Figure 2.1.

Age and gender

Age and gender correlate with health outcomes and both are easy to define and measure, but taken alone are rarely robust indicators of inequalities in health and are not modifiable factors. It is known, for example, that death rates are relatively high in children up to the age of four years and then decrease, but childhood mortality and morbidity can vary within populations. When data is standardised to the population norm and differences between areas explored, it can be demonstrated that babies born to poor families are at much greater risk of prematurity, low birth weight and infant mortality, illness, disability, injury and accidents. In fact, virtually all aspects of health are worse among children living in poverty than among those from affluent backgrounds.

Ethnicity/race

Ethnicity can be associated with a range of health and mortality issues but is often the consequence of socioeconomic differentials. In addition, the health of ethnic groups is influenced by factors such as cultural bonds, social ties, extended families and genetics. Racism, harassment and geographical/residential segregation also play a part, as may lifestyle. For example, the higher mortality among the Irish when living in England may be linked to their high alcohol consumption when compared with the English, and with the Irish in Ireland.[5]

While ethnicity may be a useful indicator for measuring potential inequalities, it needs to be combined with other socioeconomic and demographic measures to have validity. Moreover, given that different definitions for ethnicity have been used in the 1981, 1991 and 2001 Censuses in the UK, longitudinal analysis of the relationship between ethnicity, deprivation and inequalities in health can be problematic.

Modifiable factors: individual lifestyle factors

A variety of personal behaviours influence health, some examples of which are described here. (See also smoking and sexual health in Chapter 11). These determinants of health can all be found at level 4 in Figure 2.1.

Diet and weight management

The UK is experiencing one of the world's fastest growing rates of obesity and this has a direct impact on diseases such as cancer and cardiovascular disease, and leads to premature mortality and morbidity. Obesity is considered to be at epidemic proportions with almost 24% of men and women classified as obese (body mass index over 30 kg/m^2) and 25% of children aged 11–15 years of age being overweight (body mass index over 25 kg/m^2).

Being overweight can seriously affect an individual's health and may lead to high blood pressure, type 2 diabetes, cardiovascular disease, many cancers including colorectal and prostate cancers in men and breast or endometrial cancer in women, osteoarthritis, poor self image and decreased life expectancy. In general, lower socioeconomic groups in the UK are more likely to be overweight and obese and consume less fruit, vegetables, fish and wholegrain cereals and more refined foods high in fat, sugar and salt. As a consequence, these dietary patterns, coupled with weight management issues, make a significant contribution to the pattern of diseases experienced by the different socioeconomic groups.

Alcohol

Excessive alcohol intake is associated with a range of health problems, including serious liver disease, disorders of the stomach and pancreas, anxiety and depression, sexual problems, high blood pressure and cardiac disease, involvement in accidents, particularly road accidents, a range of cancers, including those of the mouth, throat, liver, colon and breast, and becoming overweight or obese.

Alcohol misuse accounts for approximately 22 000 deaths each year with consumption above the recommended limit of three units per day for men and two units per day for females being exceeded by 22% of adult females and 39% of adult males. Of particular concern is the fact that 20% of the population in England drink to get drunk (binge drink), defined as consuming more than eight units for men and six units in females, and is strongly associated with involvement in accidents and cardiovascular disease. Alcohol-related deaths are more than threefold higher in the most deprived than the least deprived sectors of society.[6]

Exercise

Regular exercise for adults that is equivalent to at least 30 minutes a day of moderate physical activity, on five or more days of the week, can help prevent or manage a range of disorders including cardiovascular disease, type 2 diabetes, musculoskeletal disorders, mental illness and a range of cancers. Children are required to undertake at least 60 minutes of moderate activity each day to promote healthy growth, development and psychological well-being. Recent surveys have shown less than 37% of adult men and 24% of women undertake sufficient exercise to gain any health benefit. Physical inactivity is twice as common for individuals in the most deprived than the least deprived socioeconomic sectors of society.

Social and economic factors

The determinants of health described here can be seen at level 3 in Figure 2.1.

Social capital

There is no widely accepted definition of social capital but the term is used to represent social organisation that acts as a resource available to individuals through membership of social networks or communities that facilitate individual and collective action. Being able to trust others, the expectation that favours will be returned and access to plenty of high quality social interaction are all important components of social capital. For example, children living in a deprived area have fewer behavioural and emotional problems if there is high attendance at church in the area and neighbourhood support schemes are in place. Individuals who enjoy living in a neighbourhood where there is high reciprocity and plenty of community activity report better self-rated health.

Economic status

Economic status and health outcomes are intimately related. The concept that there is a direct relationship between wealth and health holds in many settings but is often difficult to assess because details of income and take-home pay are often far from transparent because of different benefit and bonus systems. While taxable income is declared to the government, there is no other routine record of income. As a consequence of the need to capture details of economic status, other measures, such as car ownership and council tax band are used to indicate economic status and are incorporated into methodologies to measure deprivation.

Car ownership

The UK Census asks whether a household has one, two or more cars and can thereby express car ownership as residents in households with no car as a proportion of all residents. At one time (probably in the mid to late 1980s) car ownership was a good proxy for wealth, if not income. Nowadays car owner-ship has increased across all sectors of society. The issue of car ownership as a proxy for wealth and thereby health has been further diminished by access to company cars and a reduction in public transport in some areas, which has forced more to use private transport. In rural parts of Wales and Scotland this is often a particular problem because a car is essential for travel regardless of income. In contrast, traffic congestion and parking problems in cities cause otherwise wealthy people not to own a car.

Council tax band

Council tax band is a good indicator of property value and can be used as a proxy for income and wealth. Limitations to its use include the fact that individuals of lower income do not always live in houses of least value, while people on high incomes do not always live in high cost housing. This rela-tionship between income and tax band is further confounded by high earners with no children who choose smaller, less expensive property while the elderly may not wish to leave their large family home. Overall, council tax band represents data that can be easily captured and incorporated in methodologies to quantify deprivation but there are limitations to its sensitivity and specificity.

Social class

A classification for social class was first devised for the 1911 Census in order to group individuals according to wealth. An assessment of social class has been included in every census since but each time with some modification. The occupation-based classification used to indicate socioeconomic position in the 2001 Census was the National Statistics Socioeconomic Classification (NS-SeC) and is shown in Box 2.1.

> **Box 2.1** *National Statistics Socio-economic Classification* used to indicate socioeconomic status*
>
> *Class 1:* higher managerial and professional occupations (six subgroups)
> *Class 2:* lower managerial and professional (six subgroups)
> *Class 3:* intermediate occupations (four subgroups)
> *Class 4:* small employers and own account workers (four subgroups)
> *Class 5:* lower supervisory and technical occupations (three subgroups)
> *Class 6:* semi-routine occupations (seven subgroups)
> *Class 7:* routine occupations (five subgroups)
> *Class 8:* never worked and long term unemployed
>
> *More detail can be found on the UK government website at: http://www.ons.gov.uk/ about-statistics/classifications/current/ns-sec/index.html (accessed 20 November 2009).
>
> Source: Office for National Statistics. Crown Copyright material is reproduced with the permission of the Office of Public Sector Information (OPSI).

Despite many limitations of associations with social class, it is recognised that:

- there is a consistent gradient between occupational class and death, which increases from managerial and professional classifications to unskilled labourers and can be demonstrated in both men and women
- the occupational class of the father is associated with the chance of survival of a baby in the perinatal period, i.e. the higher the occupational class the better the outcome for the baby
- gradients exist between occupational class and both chronic and acute illness.

Family structure

Health status in adulthood is influenced by childhood experience. It is assumed the socioeconomic status of the household or parents best reflects this, but family or household structure are also important. Both have long term effects on health and are probably the consequence of biological development and social and environmental circumstances.

Among adults, married people generally have lower death rates than single or divorced persons and are less likely to report long standing chronic illness and psychiatric disorders. In the past there was a strong association between marital status and health, but the trend towards cohabitation means this is now less reliable as an indicator of inequalities in health.

Living, working and socioeconomic conditions

Living and working conditions and general socioeconomic conditions are shown at level 2 and level 1, respectively in Figure 2.1. Some of these are described here.

Employment status

Employment is an important measure of social position and generally serves as a guide to income. It is a straightforward concept but can represent a wide range of circumstances that are difficult to quantify. Typical of this would be the problem of categorising someone who works on a voluntary basis or the case of the individual who is in employment but their income is exceptionally low. Even if an individual is in employment and this provides a reasonable income, the nature of the work can have an adverse effect on well-being and the ability to stay healthy. Occupational diseases are an obvious by-product of a poor work environment because of factors such as physical and chemical exposure to lead, carbon disulphide or carbon monoxide. Job security has also been recognised as important for well-being. The trend towards less secure, short term employment affects everyone but is a particular problem for less skilled manual workers.

In addition to job security there is considerable evidence that greater control over work is associated with positive health such as a lower prevalence of coronary heart disease, fewer musculoskeletal disorders, reduced mental illness and less sickness absence. The relationship between status in the workforce and health has been demonstrated across the gradient from the top job to those at the bottom. Studies with civil servants in Whitehall, London[7,8] demonstrated that even those in the next grade down from the top had worse health than those in the top posts. Despite being in well-paid and relatively secure posts a health gradient was observed across a range of disorders when compared with those in the top posts.

Unemployment and social disadvantage are closely linked and have an impact on health. A number of the health problems that can be linked to unemployment are set out in Box 2.2. Unfortunately the link between ill

Box 2.2 *Examples of the health burden associated with unemployment*

- Increased smoking
- Increased alcohol consumption
- Reduced physical activity and exercise
- Increased use of illicit drugs
- Increased sexual risk taking and sexually transmitted diseases
- Increased weight gain
- Reduced psychological well-being, e.g. self harm, depression, anxiety
- Increased morbidity
- Increased premature mortality from diseases such as coronary heart disease
- Social exclusion and isolation

health and unemployment is not straightforward as people with poorer health are themselves more likely to be unemployed. This is particularly true for people with long term conditions although this, alone, does not fully explain why the unemployed have poorer health.

Education

Achievement in education is a good guide to social position, can easily be defined and serves as a strong indicator of inequalities in health. Moreover, educational achievements change little beyond early adulthood and are rarely influenced by subsequent illness while occupation and income can change quite markedly throughout life as a result of health problems.

Educational attainment influences inequalities in socioeconomic position and health[9] by determining the position of an individual in the labour market and the subsequent impact this has on income, housing and material possessions. Education also prepares children for a healthy life by providing them with both social and emotional knowledge and skills to help them relate to others, participate fully in society and navigate the healthcare system to their benefit.

Environment

Area of residence

In England there is a gradient from the low levels of age standardised mortality seen in the south and east of the country to the high levels of the north and west. Intriguingly this gradient exists for most common causes of death including circulatory disease, malignant neoplasm, respiratory disease, accidents, poisonings and violence. There are also variations within, as well as between, regions with the area of residence having an independent effect upon the health of individuals and households within a given area. As a consequence, place of residence can be a relatively sensitive measure of potential deprivation, inequality and need, particularly if combined with other measures of socioeconomic or demographic status. Both area of residence and housing generally reflect, rather than create, socioeconomic and health gradients.

Urban–rural setting

Living in a rural setting in the UK is often considered to be idyllic and a place where the urban wealthy have second homes. In reality it is often associated with higher levels of poverty and ill health. Psychiatric morbidity is a particular problem for dwellers in rural communities. It is, however, simplistic to assume all rural areas are the same. The health of the population in an isolated village in a remote, former mining area of south Wales with high unemployment will be different from that of a wealthy village in a southeast England commuter belt. Rurality per se is therefore not a good indicator of health.

Housing

Housing conditions can be used to highlight potential health inequalities. Poor housing, often defined in terms of overcrowding, damp and mould, indoor pollutants and infestation, cold, homelessness and the use of temporary accommodation have all been shown to have a detrimental effect on health (Table 2.1).[10] Of these factors, overcrowding is perhaps the easiest to measure as it can be calculated from the national census from data on persons in households with one or more persons per room as a proportion of all residents in households.

In the UK there is a fuel poverty strategy which seeks to provide heating and insulation improvement for those who spend 10% or more of their income on heating their home. The rationale for this is that cold homes exacerbate many existing illnesses such as asthma and make the individual

Table 2.1 The consequences of poor housing for physical health[10]	
Circumstance	**Consequence**
Overcrowding	Increased risk of infectious or respiratory disease
	Reduced stature
Damp and mould	Respiratory problems, e.g. wheezing
	Asthma, rhinitis and alveolitis
	Eczema
Indoor pollutants and infestations	Asthma
Cold	Diminished resistance to respiratory infection
	Hypothermia
	Bronchospasm
	Ischaemic heart disease, myocardial infarction and stroke
Homelessness – rooflessness	Problems resulting from facing the elements without protection
Homelessness – temporary accommodation	Problems resulting from overcrowding, noise, inadequate cooking and washing facilities
Reproduced with permission of 'South East Public Health Observatory'.	

prone to respiratory infections. In addition, fuel poverty brings opportunity loss. Poor families spend a disproportionate amount of their income to keep warm and this has an adverse effect on their social well-being, ability to adopt a healthy lifestyle and overall quality of life.

In addition to poor housing there is also evidence to suggest high rise accommodation can contribute to stress and mental health problems in adults and respiratory problems in children. This appears to be a particular problem in the UK and is less evident in other European countries where a higher percentage of the population live in high rise buildings but without the same apparent adverse effect on health. Overall the mechanism that links poor housing to ill health is not straightforward or directly causal but needs to be factored in to both the measurement of deprivation and any attempts to reduce inequalities in health.

Crime

Crime affects not only the health of the victim but also that of the community involved. Fear of crime is a real phenomenon that impacts on both health and well-being. As a consequence of crime, or the perception of crime, people make adjustments to their lifestyle and behaviour such as not going out after dark, not going out alone, avoiding certain areas, not using public transport, reducing social interaction, a general increase in mistrust and a preference to avoid young people. Because crime is often concentrated in particular neighbourhoods and the avoidance measures outlined are adopted this can weaken social ties, undermine social cohesion and have a negative impact on health. Interventions that have targeted unsafe housing estates and tried to make them more safe have resulted in a consequent improvement in health.[11]

Air quality

One of the most enduring images of poor air quality are the photographs of London in dense smog in the 1950s. At the time pollution arising from the burning of domestic coal accounted for a significant number of premature deaths among Londoners. In the London smog of 1952 there was almost a threefold increase in death in the over 65s, while deaths from bronchitis and emphysema rose more than ninefold, pneumonia and influenza increased fourfold and myocardial degeneration increased almost threefold along with associated increases in hospital admissions. Although the sulphur dioxide and black smoke from coal is now a thing of the past, other pollutants have taken their place notably from the burning of petrol and diesel from cars and other forms of transport. Ambient levels of air pollution continue to be associated with raised morbidity and mortality and are particularly hazardous to the elderly, children and those with pre-existing disease.

Measurement of deprivation

Although we cannot explain the interrelationship between the determinants of health, we can quantify a number of the contributory parameters and use them to measure deprivation, indicate inequalities in health and assist in targeting healthcare resources according to need.

There is no single, sensitive and accurate means of quantifying the factors that impact on health and result in inequalities. Problems with defining social groups and individual standing in society and health status, together with endeavours to describe and quantify the relationship between social disadvantage, are all complex and many have been outlined above. There are three broad areas that are most frequently quantified to inform the debate on inequalities:

- social demography (age, area of residence, sex and ethnicity/race)
- social and economic status (car ownership, employment, income, occupational social class, socioeconomic groupings)
- social environment (housing conditions, social networks, social support).

Townsend index

One of the most widely used measures of deprivation is the Townsend index, developed in 1988 to provide a material measure of deprivation and disadvantage. The index is based on four different variables taken, originally from the 1991 Census, namely:

- *unemployment:* percentage of economically active residents aged 16–59 (female)/16–64 (male) unemployed and excluding students
- *non-car ownership:* percentage of private households who do not possess a car or van
- *non-home ownership:* percentage of private households not owner occupied
- *household overcrowding:* percentage of private households overcrowded (more than one person per room).

These variables produce a composite score for relative deprivation. The higher the score, the more deprived and disadvantaged an area is thought to be, thereby allowing different areas to be ranked in relation to one another.

The Townsend index has a number of limitations, including lack of validity in rural areas where, unlike urban areas, ownership of a car may be a necessity at all levels of deprivation as discussed above. However, the Townsend index continues to be widely used because its construction is independent of health-related variables, the component data are captured in the national census and it permits comparison of deprivation between countries in the UK.

Carstairs score

Carstairs scores were designed as a summary measure of relative deprivation within small populations and were first calculated on data from the 1981 Census. Like the Townsend index, the Carstairs score is based on four indicators from the census. These four variables from the 2001 Census are:

- *unemployment*: unemployed males 16 and over as a proportion of all economically active males aged 16 and over
- *car ownership*: residents in households with no car as a proportion of all residents in households
- *overcrowding*: residents in households with one or more per room as a proportion of all residents in households
- *low social class*: residents in households with an economically active head of household in social class IV or V as a proportion of all residents in households.

The scores are an unweighted combination of the four census variables. After standardisation the values for each variable are summed to give a score that can be either positive (more deprived) or negative (less deprived). The limitations to the Carstairs scores are not dissimilar to the problems seen with the Townsend index. Rural deprivation may be invisible and car ownership is more of a necessity in rural areas, thereby reducing the sensitivity of the scores.

Index of multiple deprivation

The index of multiple deprivation (IMD) is a measure of multiple deprivation at the small area level. It is based on a range of domains of deprivation that can be identified and measured separately but then aggregated to give a composite score with different weightings for the different domains. An individual may be counted in one or more of the domains depending on the number of types of deprivation they experience.

Each of the 32 482 lower super output areas in England (lower layer super output areas are geographical areas designed to improve reporting of small-area statistics and relate to areas of minimum population 1000 and mean population 1500) have been assigned a score and rank for the seven domains (Table 2.2). There are also two supplementary indices: income deprivation affecting children and income deprivation affecting older people.

The IMD in England has gone through a number of changes over the years and therefore it can be problematic comparing the overall deprivation score with values compiled using previous and different methodologies. Similarly, differences occur with the calculation of the IMD in the different countries within the UK because of the use of different data sources. This variation has

Table 2.2 The seven domains of the Index of Multiple Deprivation (2007) used in England with the weighting for each domain

Domain	Weighting (%)
Income deprivation	22.5
Employment deprivation	22.5
Education, skills and training deprivation	13.5
Health deprivation and disability	13.5
Barriers to housing and services	9.3
Crime	9.3
Living environment deprivation	9.3

emerged because of the country-specific nature of the deprivation that occurs within each country. For example, the IMD in Wales has eight domains. These include income, employment, health, education, housing, access to services, physical environment and community safety. As a consequence of the different component domains and different weightings it is not possible to compare deprivation in different countries on the basis of scores from the IMD.

References

1. Decennial life tables (2000–02). *Population Trends 136*. London: Office of National Statistics, 2009. http://www.statistics.gov.uk/downloads/theme_population/PopTrends_Report.pdf (accessed 20 November 2009).
2. Department of Health and Social Security. *Inequalities in Health: Report of a research working group* (The Black Report). London: DHSS, 1980.
3. Annual report of the Chief Medical Officer, Department of Health. London: The Stationery Office, 1990.
4. Dahlgren G, Whitehead M. *Policies and Strategies to Promote Social Equity in Health*. Stockholm: Institute for Future Studies, 1991.
5. Harrison L, Carr-Hill R, Sutton M. Consumption and harm: drinking patterns of the Irish, the English and the Irish in England. *Alcohol Alcoholism* 1993; 28: 715–723.
6. Wales Centre for Health. *A Profile of Alcohol in Wales*. Cardiff: Wales Centre for Health, 2009. www.nphs.wales.nhs.uk (accessed 20 November 2009).
7. Marmot MG, Davey-Smith G, Stansfield SA *et al*. Health inequalities among British civil servants: the Whitehall II study. *Lancet* 1991; 337: 1387–1393.
8. Marmot MG, Shipley MJ, Rose G. Inequalities in death: specific explanations of a general pattern. *Lancet* 1984; 323: 1003–1006.
9. Acheson D. *Independent Inquiry into Inequalities in Health*. London: Stationery Office, 1998.
10. Carr-Hill R, Chalmers-Dixon P. *The Public Health Observatory Handbook of Health Inequalities Measurement*. Oxford: South East Public Health Observatory, 2005.
11. Halpern DS. *Mental Health and the Built Environment: More than bricks and mortar?* London: Taylor and Francis 1995.

3

Pharmacy within public health: a UK perspective

Christine M Bond and Margaret C Watson

The Faculty of Public Health was founded in 1972 by the three Royal Colleges of Physicians in the United Kingdom (London, Edinburgh and Glasgow). Initially called the Faculty of Community Medicine, it essentially represented a specialist area of medical practice designed to train and assess public health doctors. However, during the last decade, as UK policy and practice has encouraged greater interprofessional working and extension of roles, this same change has been reflected in the delivery of public health services.

Importantly, public health is recognised as 'reaching far beyond the usual confines of NHS structures'[1] and thus, as well as roles in the NHS, it encompasses roles in national and local government agencies, notably military, community and voluntary organisations and academia. It draws on a wide spectrum of disciplinary expertise, including other healthcare professionals such as pharmacists, dentists and nurses, health promotion specialists, as well as health economists, statisticians, information scientists and many more.

A further recent change in the way public health is delivered is an awareness that while for some people – referred to as public health specialists – all, or virtually all, of their remit will be about public health, for others, such as pharmacists employed in more traditional roles in community, primary and secondary care, public health, or contributing to improving health, it is but one component of a role that has many other elements. Those engaged in public health in this latter role have recently been labelled as working in public health or public health practitioners.[2] This chapter provides an overview of the sort of activities pharmacists are engaged in as either specialists or practitioners. Many of the topics are revisited in detail in other chapters. It also provides an overview of the training, career progression and continuing professional development requirements of engaging in public health work.

The public health role can be broken down in a number of different ways. One of the simplest frameworks, which is also of relevance to pharmacy,[3] identifies three domains of public health practice: health protection and prevention, health and social care and health improvement (see Box 1.1 in Chapter 1).

The 10 core elements of practice originally developed by the Faculty of Public Health and adopted by other organisations, including the DoH, cut across these three domains, and are the basis of competency assessments, such as those listed in Box 3.1.

Box 3.1 *The 10 core elements of public health practice (from PharmacyHealthLink[4])*

1   Surveillance and assessment of the population's health and well-being
2   Promoting and protecting the population's health and well-being
3   Developing quality and risk management within an evaluative culture
4   Collaboratively working for health
5   Developing health programmes and services and reducing inequalities
6   Policy and strategy development and implementation
7   Working with and for communities
8   Strategic leadership for health and well-being
9   Research and development to improve health and well-being
10   Ethically managing self, people and resources to improve health and well-being

Reproduced with permission of PH link (www.pharmacyhealth.link.org.uk)

Pharmacists as public health practitioners

While pharmacists are employed at all levels outlined in Chapter 1, they also work in different settings. The following sections describe some of the public health activities pharmacists can and do engage in at a practitioner level, as part of their daily work in primary and secondary care.

Primary care

Community pharmacy

Historically, community pharmacists have always had a health promotion role but this has been expanded over recent years to become more proactive in terms of health improvement. While the greater focus on public health involvement and extended roles in community pharmacy has generated controversy[5] and concerns about being a diversion from the 'medicines expert' role of pharmacists,[6] there is growing recognition among healthcare planners and policy makers of the contribution that community pharmacists, pharmacists and pharmacy support staff can make to public health. The evidence of and for this contribution has been compiled in substantial reviews[7–9] and demonstrates the breadth of public health activities and services that can be and are provided in community pharmacies and/or by community pharmacists and their staff.

In 2005, the DoH in England issued its strategy for pharmaceutical public health for the next 10 years, *Choosing Health through Pharmacy*.[10] The strategy identifies public health priorities, the targets for addressing them, and the contribution that pharmacy can make to meeting these targets. Public health is now one of the seven essential services required of community pharmacy contractors in England, through the community pharmacy contractual framework for England and Wales. This requires pharmacists to provide opportunistic healthy lifestyle advice to certain populations presenting prescriptions and to promote public health messages during targeted campaigns. Similarly, in Scotland, the community pharmacy contract comprises a public health component[11] which includes general public health activities and participation in campaigns, as well as specific public health services, e.g. smoking cessation, emergency hormonal contraception. Although different national strategies, policies and/or contracts for each of the home countries exist, the general tenets of each are similar. In terms of health protection and prevention, many pharmacy-based services are already provided in community pharmacies throughout the UK (Box 3.2).

Box 3.2 *Examples of health protection and prevention services provided by community pharmacies*

- Disposal of waste medicines
- Flu vaccination clinics
- Travel health clinics
- Methadone maintenance
- Needle exchange services
- Sexual health services – emergency hormonal contraception, sexually transmitted infections/HIV testing, free condoms
- Smoking cessation services
- Healthy weight management
- Patient safety – pharmacovigilance
- Head lice treatment

In terms of health and social care, community pharmacists and their staff may contribute to the efficient use of medicines through a variety of activities, which support medicines use in individual patients. The community pharmacy contractual framework for England and Wales, introduced in April 2005, also included 'clinical governance' as one of the specified essential services. Clinical governance activities related to patient safety include maintenance of a log of patient safety incidents, standard operating procedures, participation in audit, managing and training staff, continuing professional development and use of information. In relation to health improvement activities, community pharmacies and pharmacists can make considerable contributions, particularly in terms of inequalities, education and healthy lifestyles. A case study of how pharmacists can address inequalities is presented in Box 3.3.

Box 3.3 *Case study: needs assessment of pharmaceutical care – the Middlefield Project*

The Middlefield Project is an example of a pharmaceutical service that was developed as the result of a needs assessment of pharmaceutical care. Middlefield is an area in Aberdeen city which had a high level of deprivation. In terms of public health, this area had a high prevalence of heart and respiratory diseases, as well as mental health problems. The population of 3500 was not served by a general practice or a community pharmacy. The 'Healthy Hoose' was established as an outreach health service to address some of the health needs of the community but did not originally include pharmaceutical care services. Therefore, in 2001, a needs assessment was undertaken to identify priorities for pharmaceutical care service provision. Full details of this assessment are available.[12] Based on the results of the assessment, a novel pharmaceutical service was developed and established in the Healthy Hoose, consisting of a part-time community pharmacy service for the provision of advice on minor illness and advice and sale (or supply) of over-the-counter medicines. In addition, the pharmacist was able to provide direct supply of a range of medicines from a defined formulary, to patients who were exempt from prescription charges. The evaluation of the first year of the service demonstrated the wide range of pharmaceutical services provided to and accessed by the population in Middlefield[13] including the treatment of head lice, smoking cessation advice and treatment, as well as prescription collection. This case study demonstrates how the need for pharmaceutical services can be identified and services developed to meet the needs of the population, in this case, a deprived population with inequity of access to other health services, including community pharmacy services.

A second case study is presented in Box 3.4, which describes the contribution that pharmacists can make to healthy lifestyle through providing healthy weight management services. Community pharmacies can function as health information centres, i.e. the provision of health information/advice/ materials (e.g. free condoms), as well as through pharmacists actively engaging with the community served by the pharmacy, e.g. general public, schools, other local health professionals.

Box 3.4 *Case study: weight management service provided by a community pharmacy*

Several services and studies have been conducted in the community pharmacy setting to evaluate weight management support. One of these services, provided in Coventry, England, was presented as an example of 'Pharmacy in Action' by the Royal Pharmaceutical Society of Great Britain (RPSGB).[14] The service was developed as a result of high levels of obesity in the city: 52 000 obese adults (total population approximately 306 000). The pharmacy-based service was developed by the Primary Care Trust (PCT) and offered help to adults whose body mass index was between 30 and 38 kg/m^2 and who had a minimum of one additional risk factor for heart disease or type 2 diabetes. Ten pharmacies provided the weight management service initially, with more joining the scheme thereafter. The service included an initial consultation with a pharmacist followed by the provision of materials (e.g. diary, information booklet) and the setting of goals for weight loss. The results from the pilot study showed that over two thirds of patients lost weight and nearly three quarters of patients reduced their waist circumference. This is an example of a health improvement service that could be provided in most community pharmacies to promote and achieve lifestyle change, particularly in patients who are at risk from serious or chronic disease.

Practice pharmacy

Primary care pharmacists will increasingly find opportunities in both primary care organisations and/or at regional level to influence local pharmacy strategy development, working increasingly with the specialist pharmacists in pharmaceutical public health who have chosen to make public health pharmacy their discipline. In terms of health protection and prevention, practice pharmacists (as with all pharmacists working in clinical settings) can contribute to patient safety in terms of pharmacovigilance as part of medication reviews and in reporting adverse reactions. They can also contribute to reducing the volume of waste medicines, thus reducing the risk of environmental health hazards associated with unused medicines. In terms of health and social care, practice pharmacists can promote quality prescribing among their general practitioner (GP) colleagues and provide an educational role in ensuring that their primary care colleagues are informed about new evidence of clinical effectiveness, for example, the treatment of long term conditions.

Practice pharmacists who have prescribing rights can further contribute to public health by ensuring prescribed medicines for patients with long term conditions are appropriate and comply with evidence-based recommendations. During medication reviews and other contacts with patients, practice pharmacists can provide educational materials and advice about healthy lifestyles, and signpost or refer patients to appropriate services, e.g. smoking cessation or weight management.

Secondary care

Hospital pharmacy has a role in secondary prevention and an integrated approach to service provision. At a population level pharmacists have traditional roles in drug information and advice on effective medication usage. In secondary care, pharmacists also play an important public health role and examples can be found illustrating their contribution to each of the three core domains. Again this chapter provides examples, rather than a comprehensive list of all possible public health activities.

One of pharmacists' biggest public health roles in secondary care is their contribution to patient safety through the detection and resolution of medication-related errors. Ideally this should occur before the patient is affected. In most UK hospitals, specialist clinical pharmacists review patients' medication records on a daily basis, identifying and correcting prescribing errors. They also contribute to checking safe medication recording and administration by nurses and doctors.

Related to safe medication use is the pharmacist's role in pharmacovigilance. The Yellow Card Scheme (YCS)[15] was introduced in the UK in 1964, following the thalidomide disaster (see Chapter 14). It provides a system to collect information on suspected adverse drug reactions to medicines as part of an 'early warning' or signal generation system. The scheme was initially only for the use of doctors, but hospital pharmacy reporting was introduced in 1997. A key role for public health pharmacy is to increase pharmacist reporting to both the national YCS and also to develop local databases on patient safety.

Pharmacists are key personnel in the hospital setting. Their traditional roles in maintaining supply of quality medicines, ensuring appropriate storage of products, and checking their expiry dates remain important functions. In their increasingly recognised role as expert advisers in medicines, they also play a vital and often leading part on hospital drug and therapeutic committees and formulary committees (see Chapter 14). Their systematic approach to reviewing evidence is often called upon when assessing new drugs, drawing on evidence published by national bodies such as NICE, the Scottish Intercollegiate Guidelines Network (SIGN) and the Scottish Medicines Consortium (SMC).

Pharmacists also play their part in audit and governance around the use of medicines, including adherence to national and local guidelines, to ensure drugs are only prescribed and administered in accordance with the most up to date evidence.[16]

There are also health improvement opportunities for pharmacists in the hospital setting. The increasing contact pharmacists have with patients means they are well placed, in common with all other health professionals, to reinforce healthy lifestyle messages to patients especially around smoking, diet and alcohol consumption. Many hospitals now have more streamlined approaches for continuity of pharmaceutical care at both admission and discharge, of particular relevance for people engaged in smoking cessation attempts initiated in either setting. Similarly, especially at discharge, pharmacists provide individual patients with advice on the appropriate use of their medicines, including how to store them and take them. This has benefit both for inpatient use of medicines and educationally in the longer term.

Other

Academic pharmacy

In academia, research and teaching pharmaceutical public health is similarly a growing area of development across the UK. Academia supports the evidence base for future practice and ensures that tomorrow's practitioners are both pharmacists and public health practitioners.

To be a registered pharmacist in the UK, all pharmacists must have successfully completed an undergraduate masters-level degree programme at a school of pharmacy accredited by the Royal Pharmaceutical Society of Great Britain (RPSGB). The schools are required to deliver a curriculum based on an indicative syllabus[17] which includes 51 areas of study, of which one is specifically labelled 'public health and the role of the pharmacist'. A further 10 areas are of relevance to the public health agenda, such as 'drug and substance misuse' and 'clinical evaluation of new and existing drugs'.

However, it is not only in teaching all potential pharmacists about public health topics where academia can contribute. Many schools of pharmacy and other university centres have increasing interest in health services research applied to pharmacy, often referred to as pharmacy practice research. Evidence derived from these studies has informed the development of services subsequently rolled out to the wider workforce, such as smoking cessation advice from community pharmacies[18,19] and detecting and reducing medication errors in secondary care.[20]

Pharmaceutical industry

The pharmaceutical industry must target research and development to reflect national health priorities and work in partnership with healthcare providers to ensure best use of available resources. This is happening already as clinical trials increasingly include cost-effectiveness data to inform health technology assessments. It is also the industry's responsibility to contribute to pharmacovigilance, for example, with the YCS, as suspected adverse drug reactions are reported via companies' medical information departments (see Chapter 14). A better partnership between the industry and the NHS has also been encouraged recently, with greater openness and sharing of pre-marketing information to add to the evidence base considered by the new drugs review processes carried out by organisations such as the SMC and NICE.

Pharmacist public health specialists

Specialist pharmacists are employed to provide pharmacy-related strategic input into public health decision making and, reciprocally, public health input into strategic pharmacy decision making at health boards (Scotland, Wales and Northern Ireland) and at the level of primary care organisations and at regional level in England. In both Scotland and Wales, the role is well established, with a specialist in pharmaceutical public health in post in nearly all health boards, as well as special health boards such as Health Protection Scotland, the Information Statistics Division (Scotland) and Public Health Wales. The following sections are, as before, not intended to be exhaustive but are indicative of the scope of activity with which pharmacists can become involved. Pharmacists employed in specialist areas such as Health Protection Scotland, will operate within a more limited, but more in-depth remit.

Within health protection there are many examples of the types of areas to which pharmaceutical public health can contribute. At the time of writing, the H1N1 influenza pandemic is an excellent example of the need to have pharmacy input into the supply and administration of both antivirals and vaccines. Indeed pharmacists have a leading role in all immunisation programmes, overlapping with their role in service planning and the use of community pharmacists to both promote uptake of vaccines and to administer them directly. Other areas of relevance where pharmacy input is important in health protection include drug misuse, appropriate use of medicines, distribution and monitoring of drug alerts (see Chapters 12 and 14) and emergency planning of pharmacy services in the event of a pandemic or bioterrorism.

Pharmacists are also increasingly involved in medicines management at area and national levels through their lead role on area wide committees reviewing evidence for the introduction of new drugs and equitable allocation of resources across a population (see Chapter 14). With respect to other key areas of work in this domain, they often play a part in implementing new guidelines and standards, especially those where pharmacological intervention is a major component. They also often ensure compliance with regulations. For example, the specialist in pharmaceutical public health is mandated within the Patient Group Directions (PGD) guidance[21] to ensure that those operating within PGD regulatory frameworks are adequately trained and monitored.

Service planning is also very much part of the specialist's day to day work; they identify local area targets where pharmacy could contribute to achieving the delivered outcomes such as delivery of travel medicines,[22] palliative care supplies and treatment, near patient testing schemes, out-of-hours care. Operating within a public health framework means that these services can be developed systematically following well-conducted needs assessment, review of the national and international evidence, and consideration of the likely cost/benefit balance (see Chapters 6–9).

Many of the pharmacy roles within health improvement, such as smoking cessation, reduced alcohol intake, better diet and obesity targeted interventions, have already been mentioned as relating to community pharmacists (see Chapter 11). However, at an organisational level, the specialist in pharmaceutical public health provides overarching coordination to develop, implement, monitor and evaluate the schemes. They also can devise new ways of addressing inequalities,[12] again overlapping with service planning or providing community-based education and input into schools.

Training

To become a specialist in pharmaceutical public health requires a formal approach. To be taken seriously as fully fledged colleagues in the public health team, an equivalent qualification to the consultant in public health medicine has to be achieved. The latter follow similar training to other medical specialities, i.e. five years of specialist training after two foundation years of postgraduation practice. When pharmacists first became engaged at this level there was exploration of dual registration with the Faculty of Public Health and the Royal Pharmaceutical Society of Great Britain (RPSGB), in much the same way that consultants in dental public health train. However, these initial developments were superseded by the establishment of the UK Public Health Register (UKPHR) often referred to as the 'Voluntary Register', which brings together registration for specialists in public health and has routes for medically and dentally qualified applicants, as well as other disciplines with extensive experience of public health but less formal training. These latter individuals achieve registration by successful completion of a portfolio-based assessment which can be badged as either a 'specialist status' (sometimes referred to as generalist) or 'defined specialist status'. The portfolios cover the domains and core areas of public health practice listed previously (see Boxes 1.1 and 3.1) and require applicants to submit detailed evidence demonstrating they 'know how' to deliver and 'show how' they have delivered activities reflecting the core competencies.

The portfolio route to registration was initially introduced to provide formal recognition of the status of those already working in senior positions in public health. In January 2009, a development portfolio assessment, for training of defined specialists from a less senior position, was introduced. It consists of a series of portfolio assessments completed successively until full competence in each area is demonstrated.

There is currently no formal qualification for pharmacists to operate at a public health practitioner level; however, recognising the growing interest in practitioner status, the UKPHR is currently consulting on formal recognition of the practitioner grade, again through a portfolio approach. Pharmacists on the UKPHR register are also recognised by the Faculty of Public Health and can apply to be fellows of the faculty. In addition, a UK-wide public health career and skills framework has been developed (see Chapter 1), the implementation of which aims to strengthen the capacity and capability of the public health workforce and also inform regulation through the UKPHR. Some specific roles may need accreditation; for example, to provide smoking cessation or emergency hormonal contraception services, pharmacists and their staff are required to have undertaken specific short training courses and to attend for 'refresher' training as requested. This is important to ensure that services delivered from pharmacies are of the highest standard and at least as well delivered as from other providers. An initiative started in North West England and being rolled out throughout England, the Harmonisation of Accreditation Group (HAG),[23] ensures that accredited pharmacists can move between organisational areas.

Once qualified, continuing professional development is an essential way to maintain competences and to demonstrate. The RPSGB online professional development system can be used for this purpose, as long as written confirmation is provided by the RPSGB to the UKPHR.

Career progression

To date, career progression for those in public health has probably been serendipitous and opportunistic. The career routes of current incumbents in specialist pharmaceutical public health posts are almost as many as the number of post holders, although a pattern may now begin to emerge. Those with an advanced interest at the practitioner level are well qualified for the increasing opportunities at a 'mid career' level often associated with one particular area of practice. Thus, for example, specialist pharmacists in substance misuse, and smoking cessation coordinator posts filled by pharmacists provide excellent on-the-job training in many of the public health competencies, and there are examples of people in these positions moving on to full specialist in pharmaceutical public health roles. In the future a more planned approach may be required, and the proposed developmental portfolio route to registration as a defined specialist would be an important component of career progression, but would need a national strategic approach to funding training positions. This may ultimately be provided through the Skills for Health framework,[24] but, until this is in place, the current non-systematic route remains the only option.

In summary, the pharmacy profession has fully embraced the new opportunities provided from the NHS paradigm shift from being a 'national illness service' to a 'national wellness service'. With the growing burden of an increasingly elderly UK population and the potential increase in workload associated with the management of, often self-inflicted, chronic disease, health promotion and preventing ill health developing have become key priorities. This chapter has provided an overview of how pharmacy can play a key part in making this a reality.

References

1. Faculty of Public Health (2009). *Public Health: Specialise in the bigger issue.* London: Faculty of Public Health. http://www.publichealthconferences.org.uk/careers/downloads/ph_careers_booklet.pdf (accessed 21 October 2009).
2. Faculty of Public Health (2009). *About Practitioner Development.* London: Faculty of Public Health. http://www.fphm.org.uk/prof_standards/practitioner_development/about/default.asp (accessed 21 October 2009).
3. Royal Pharmaceutical Society of Great Britain. *Public Health. A practical guide for community pharmacists.* London: RPSGB, 2004.
4. PharmacyHealthLink (2009). *PharmacyHealthLink home page.* http://www.pharmacyhealthlink.org.uk/ (accessed 29 September 2009).
5. Purkiss R, Stephens M, Pike H. Is public health the right direction for pharmacy? *Br J Clin Pharm* 2009; 1: 146–147.
6. Hassell K. Why you must focus on being experts on medicines or risk losing your way. *Pharm J* 2009; 2: 83–96.
7. Anderson C, Blenkinsopp A, Armstrong M. *The Contribution of Community Pharmacy to Improving the Public's Health. Report 1. Evidence from the peer-reviewed literature 1990–2001.* London: PharmacyHealthLink/RPSGB; 2003. Report No. 1.
8. Blenkinsopp A, Anderson C, Armstrong M. *The Contribution of Community Pharmacy to Improving the Public's Health. Report 2. Evidence from the UK non peer-reviewed literature 1990–2002.* London: PharmacyHealthLink/RPSGB; 2003. Report No.: 2.
9. Blenkinsopp A, Anderson C, Armstrong M. *The Contribution of Community Pharmacy to Improving the Public's Health. Summary report of the literature review 1990–2007.* London: PharmacyHealthLink, 2009. http://www.phlink.org.uk/files/Evidence%20Base%20Report%207.pdf.
10. Department of Health. *Choosing Health through Pharmacy.* London: Department of Health; 2005.

11. Community Pharmacy (2009). *Public Health Service*. NHS Scotland. http://www.communitypharmacy.scot.nhs.uk/core_services/phs.html (accessed 30 September 2009).
12. Porteous T, Bond C. Novel provision of pharmacy services to a deprived area: a pharmaceutical needs assessment. *IJPP* 2003; 11(47): 54.
13. King M, McFarlane K, Juroszek L *et al.* The Middlefield project: novel provision of pharmacy services to a deprived city area. *Pharm J* 2005; 275: 164–166.
14. Sharma M. Pharmacists help fight obesity in Coventry. London: RPSGB; 2008.
15. Yellow Card Scheme. http://yellowcard.mhra.gov.uk/ (accessed 30 September 2009).
16. Kamyar M, Johnson J, McAnaw J *et al.* Adherence to clinical guidelines in the prevention of coronary heart disease in type II diabetes mellitus. *Pharm World Sci* 2007; 30: 120–127.
17. Pharmacy syllabus. http://www.rpsgb.org/pdfs/edmpharmidicsyllabus.pdf (accessed 17 August 2008).
18. Sinclair HK, Bond CM, Stead LF. Community pharmacy personnel interventions for smoking cessation. *The Cochrane Library* 2004; (1).
19. Sinclair HK, Bond CM, Lennox A *et al.* Training pharmacists and pharmacy assistants in the stage-of-change model of smoking cessation: a randomised controlled trial. *Tob Control* 1998; 7: 253–261.
20. Dean B, Barber N, Schachter M. What is a prescribing error? *Qual Health Care* 2000; 9: 232–237.
21. Patient Group Directions. NHS HDL 2001/7 http://www.sehd.scot.nhs.uk/mels/HDL2001 _07.htm (accessed 21 October 2009).
22. Hind CA, Bond CM, Lee AJ *et al.* Needs assessment study of Community Travel Medicines Service. *J Travel Med* 2008; 15(5): 328–334.
23. NHS Primary Care Commissioning. Harmonisation of Accreditation Group. http://www.pcc.nhs.uk/200.php.
24. Skills for Health Framework. http://www.skillsforhealth.org.uk (accessed 6 October 2010).

Suggested reading

Hill A, Griffiths S, Gillam S. *Public Health and Primary Care: Partners in population health*. Oxford: OUP, 2007.
Donaldson LJ, Scally G. *Donaldsons' Essential Public Health*. Oxford: Radcliffe, 2009.
Orme J, Powell J, Taylor P, Grey M. *Public Health for the 21st Century: New perspectives on policy, participation and practice*. Milton Keynes: Open University, 2007.
Naidoo J, Wills J. *Public Health and Health Promotion: Developing practice*. London: Bailliere Tindall, 2004.
Health Protection Agency. *Health Emergency Planning: A handbook for practitioners*. The Stationery Office, 2008.
Graham H. *Understanding Health Inequalities*. Milton Keynes: Open University, 2009.

4

Public health data

Janet Krska and Penelope A Phillips-Howard

Information about the health of populations is necessary to identify public health problems which need attention and also to assess the effectiveness of public health interventions. The information provides a picture of a population's heath and the determinants of their health. Public health intelligence involves the collection and analysis of data from a range of sources on a continuous, repeat or ad hoc basis. These include demographic data, epidemiological data and data from surveillance.

Causality

One purpose of gathering data is to identify and measure factors that influence or cause an outcome (event, disease or death). Factors can predispose, precipitate, modify, enable or reinforce a disease, condition or disability. Outcomes may be caused by a sequence or combination of these factors or causes. Causes can be distinguished as necessary, sufficient or probable conditions. If a necessary condition can be identified and controlled, the harmful outcome can be avoided. Causes may be necessary or sufficient (or both) to result in a disease or an event. A series of nine factors, known as the Bradford-Hill criteria,[1] are used to assess evidence and guide decision making on causality (Box 4.1).

Demographic data

Demography is the statistical study of populations and the interaction of issues such as fertility, morbidity and mortality, how these are distributed by age and gender, and layered by socioeconomic and geographical determinants. To inform public health, information about lifestyle is also required. This information is gathered through a variety of techniques but must be expressed in standard ways to be useful for evaluating and comparing temporal (e.g. through longitudinal monitoring) and spatial (e.g. between geographies) trends.

> **Box 4.1** *Bradford-Hill criteria for causality assessment*
>
> *Strength:* a small association does not mean that there is not a causal effect.
> *Consistency:* the likelihood of an effect is strengthened by evidence of consistent findings observed by different people in different places with different samples.
> *Specificity:* the more specific an association between a factor and an effect, the greater the probability of a causal relationship. Causation is likely if there is no other explanation for a specific disease or outcome in a specific population at a specific place.
> *Temporality:* the effect must occur after the cause, this includes lag times or delays if these are biologically expected and plausible.
> *Biological gradient:* the larger the exposure the larger the effect, although sometimes the presence of the factor (regardless of the extent of exposure) is sufficient to trigger the effect, while alternatively the reverse may occur in some instances with greater exposure leading to a lower incidence.
> *Plausibility:* plausible mechanisms between cause and effect contribute to evidence, although limits to knowledge may diminish this.
> *Coherence:* agreement between different disciplines (e.g. laboratory and epidemiological), but differences should not nullify the epidemiological effect on associations.
> *Experiment:* experimental evidence can contribute towards knowledge of causality.
> *Analogy:* the effect of similar factors may be considered.

Data about a population can be based on:

- geography, e.g. country, regions within a country, area covered by a PCT, population registered with a particular medical practice, population served by a community pharmacy
- demographic subgroup, e.g. by age such as schoolchildren, adolescents, the elderly
- client group, e.g. users of specific services such as GP attendees, residents in nursing homes
- individual health problem, e.g. patients with diabetes, mental illness.

Data on vital events (e.g. births, deaths), use of health services and morbidity are collected locally in the UK by NHS trusts and local government organisations, nationally by the DoH, HPA and other organisations, and internationally by the European Union, Organisation for Economic Co-operation and Development (OECD) and the WHO.

Measures of health and disease

An appreciation of the ways in which health, morbidity and mortality are measured is essential to understanding these data.

Vital statistics

Data on deaths, births, marriages, stillbirths, abortions, adoptions and divorces are collected by register offices in most countries. Dates and places of birth and death, social class and occupation may be recorded. Cause of death is also usually recorded via death certificates, but is less reliable in countries without strong infrastructural support, although it is used as the source of information about disease-specific death rates. The information is supplemented by census data (see page 54) to produce an overall picture of a population. This is expressed as a pyramid in which the age and sex distribution are graphically displayed with age in the vertical axis, males on one side and females on the other (Figure 4.1). The shape of the pyramid differs particularly for populations with predominantly young (e.g. China) and

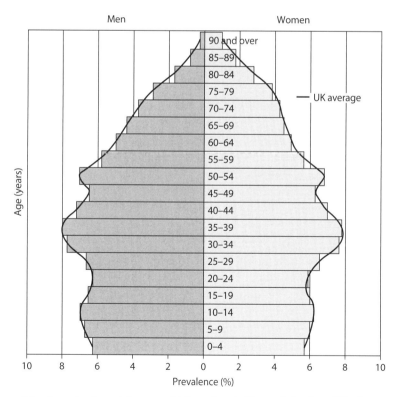

Figure 4.1 Example of population pyramid. Reproduced with permission from Office for National Statistics. Census 2001. London: ONS, 2009. Available at: http://www.statistics.gov.uk/census2001/pyramids/pages/UK.asp.[2]

old (e.g. the UK) members and characteristic differences are also apparent between low or middle income and higher income countries.

Measures of mortality

Many of the measures of mortality are ratios, requiring a numerator and a denominator. It can be difficult in some circumstances to obtain either a reliable numerator or a reliable denominator. Some ratios are expressed as annual rates and as a rate for a given number of the population, such as for every 1000 or 100 000. The simplest measure is the *mortality rate* or *crude death rate*, which is the number of deaths occurring in a specified population (derived from death registers), divided by the total population (usually derived from census data), within a set period, usually a year. The mortality rate from specific causes can also be calculated. Cause-specific death rates are usually expressed as an annual rate, for example, for lung cancer it may be 54.2 deaths per 100 000 population in a particular year.

Crude death rates will differ depending on the age distribution within a population. A young population is likely to have a lower crude death rate than an older population, since older people are more likely to die. This makes direct comparisons of crude rates between populations somewhat meaningless. Since age is a major determinant of mortality, a more refined approach is to calculate mortality rates for a population broken down by age. The most common age-specific death rate in widespread use is that for infant mortality – deaths occurring in those aged one year or less.

The *standard mortality ratio* (SMR) takes account of the age distribution of a population, so is more appropriate for comparing populations, time periods or geographical areas. It is arrived at by comparing age and sex-specific death rates for a known 'standard' population to an actual population and is expressed as a number.

$$SMR = observed\ deaths/expected\ deaths \times 100$$

If the SMR is greater than 100, then the death rate is higher than that in the comparator population. Clearly the SMR only gives relative information and is not a mortality rate, so cannot be used to describe the actual mortality rate within the population. A similar technique can be used to compare deaths in hospitals – the *hospital standard mortality ratio*. This provides evidence to determine whether the death rate in a given hospital is higher or lower than expected and is now available for most NHS hospitals in England.

Life expectancy at birth is the average number of years that members of a population born in the same year (commonly called a birth cohort) are expected to live, assuming that mortality remains constant for each age group at the time the life-expectancy is calculated. The most recent life-expectancy estimate (2010) is 66.5 years for the world population and has increased dramatically in recent years but this of course differs between countries. Overall UK life expectancy at birth is 77.4 years for males and 81.6 for females, assuming mortality rates for 2006–8.[3] It is highest in England and lowest in Scotland. As mortality rates improve, the life expectancy of the population will increase correspondingly. While the overall gap between males and females is narrowing, there are also important differences depending on socioeconomic status. For example, in Liverpool, life expectancy for males is eight years higher among those living in areas of least deprivation compared with those living in areas of highest deprivation.

Life tables can be used to calculate a relative risk of death and make demographic predictions about populations. These are often used in clinical studies, where the process can be described as survival analysis. A life table is constructed which provides data for a given population showing how many have died at given time intervals, such as a year, and also how many are left. The probability of dying within in each year is then calculated as:

$$\text{Probability} = \frac{\text{number of people dying during the year}}{\text{number alive at start of year} - (\text{number dying}/2)}$$

The probability of surviving is then 1 minus the probability of dying and the overall probability of an individual surviving the whole study or time period is calculated by multiplying the probabilities of surviving each year.

Another useful measure is the PYLL index – *potential years life lost*. This is a measure of premature mortality. It can be calculated for any age group of the population for any disease or specific cause of death, such as accidents. The calculation uses a standard life expectancy which may differ depending on the population being studied, often set at 70. The index is particularly well suited to demonstrating the impact of conditions that result in death in young people, such as childhood leukaemia.

$$\text{PYLL} = \frac{\text{sum of deaths in subgroup of population} \times (\text{life expectancy of population})}{\text{total population at risk}}$$

The burden of disease at global level can be examined using YLL data for each country, with subdivision by cause, age, sex and economic group. This provides an opportunity for comparison between countries, regions or economic group, and facilitates projections of future trends.[4] Application of potential changes, such as widespread coverage of anti-retroviral drugs, enables modelling of predicted outcomes and projected changing trends.

In the UK, as in many other countries, PYLL is on a downward trend, having decreased from 6263 in 1960 to 2564 in 2007 in females and from

9912 to 4220 over the same period in males, based on a life expectancy of 70. Some countries have a much higher PYLL, such as Mexico – 8528 in 2006 in males – while in others it is lower, for example, 3191 in Swedish males.[5]

Measures of morbidity

Two rates are used: *incidence* and *prevalence*. The incidence rate is a direct estimate of the risk of developing a disease. It can be obtained from prospective observational studies and routine data collected during surveillance. Incidence is the number of new cases occurring in a population over time. An example is the annual incidence of diabetes which is the number of newly diagnosed cases identified in the whole population over a one year period. The incidence of diabetes in the UK increased from 2.71/1000 person-years in 1996 to 4.42/1000 person-years in 2005.

$$\text{Incidence} = \frac{\text{number of new cases of a disease during a specified time period}}{\text{number of people exposed to risk of developing disease during same period}} \times 1000$$

Prevalence measures the number of cases present at any given period of time, so is calculated as:

$$\text{Prevalence} = \frac{\text{number of cases of disease present in population at a specified time}}{\text{number of people at risk of the disease at that time}} \times 1000$$

Prevalence can be point or period prevalence. The former is the number of cases at a moment in time, while the latter is over a specified period of time. Prevalence can also be calculated as the incidence of a disease multiplied by its average duration:

$$\text{Prevalence} = \text{Incidence} \times \text{Duration}$$

So for a short-lived disease which has a high incidence, such as influenza, the prevalence will usually be low, but for a long term, chronic disease, such as multiple sclerosis, despite a relatively low incidence, there will be a high prevalence, i.e. the total number of people suffering from the disease at any one time. As the incidence of a condition rises, so does the prevalence. Diabetes prevalence in the UK increased from 2.8% in 1996 to 4.3% in 2005 and the increase is associated with an increase in the prevalence of contributing risk factors such as obesity and overweight. Data on prevalence is usually gathered through surveys (see page 54). However, for cancer, there are voluntary specific registers in the UK, which monitor trends on the incidence, prevalence and also survival of patients with cancer (UK Association of Cancer Registries). The registers are used to evaluate the effectiveness of screening programmes and are used to conduct epidemiological studies of the impact of environmental and social factors on cancer risk.

Data on patients includes the site and type of cancer and is later matched with death certification to provide information about survival.

Neither prevalence nor incidence provides adequate intelligence on the burden (impact) of disease on the population, because each disease impacts differently. A measure developed for this purpose by the WHO is the *disability-adjusted life-year* (DALY), which combines morbidity and mortality data. The DALY uses PYLL, together with *years lived with disability* (YLD). One DALY is equivalent to one year of healthy life lost (either through disability or early death) and is calculated as:

$$DALY = YLL + YLD$$

YLL is calculated as the number of deaths multiplied by the standard life expectancy at age of death and YLD as the number of cases of a condition, multiplied by the average duration of the condition (from onset to death) and a disability weighting factor. This factor must be included to weight the disability which the condition creates. It is measured on a scale from 0 to 1. Using DALYs to measure disease burden modifies the relative impact of a disease. Therefore, while the leading cause of death worldwide is cardiovascular disease, comparison using DALYs places mental health as the leading cause of disability. Projected trends in global disease burdens also utilise DALYs; these suggest unipolar depressive disorders, ischaemic heart disease, Alzheimer's and other dementias, alcohol-use disorders, and diabetes will be the top five diseases of high income countries by 2030.[4]

Measures of prescribing

Prescribing data can act as a surrogate for measures of morbidity, since prescribing patterns will in general reflect disease patterns. This is limited by the extent to which specific medicines are available to treat different illnesses. Prescribing data can however, also be compared between areas within countries and between countries to generate or investigate hypotheses about factors and diseases in the same way as other types of data. Prescribing data is covered more extensively in Chapter 14.

Measures of health

Health can be measured in a variety of ways, but within public health it is most commonly measured as health-related quality of life (HRQoL). A variety of measures have been developed for use in the general population, designed to calculate a single value for current health status. Those most frequently used are probably the EuroQoL-5D (EQ-5D) and SF-36. Each method asks people about different aspects of their life, hence they are not directly comparable.

The EQ-5D consists of five dimensions (mobility, self care, usual activities, pain/discomfort, anxiety/depression) with three responses for each, plus a 20 cm visual analogue scale, designed to measure an individual's rating for their current health-related quality of life state. Weighted scores are produced giving an overall score ranging between 0 (worst health) and 1 (best health). Predictably, population norms within the UK show that overall weighted scores decrease with increasing age and significant differences occur between socioeconomic and educational groups. One advantage of the EQ-5D is that it can be used within economic studies to assess the cost-effectiveness of interventions (see Chapter 7).

The SF-36 is a multi-purpose, short-form health survey with 36 questions yielding an 8-scale profile of functional health and well-being scores. It also generates a psychometrically based physical and mental health summary measure and a preference-based health utility index. It is useful in surveys of general and specific populations, compares the relative burden of diseases and it differentiates the health benefits from different treatments.

Segmentation

To define subpopulations at risk of ill health, classification into smaller sub-groups of people according to certain characteristics is necessary. Public health data may be arranged simply by geography – for example, local government ward or PCT area. The geographical groupings now used most frequently in England and Wales are termed *output areas* (OAs) the smallest areas for which 2001 Census results are released. OAs are based on postcodes and fit within 2003 ward boundaries. There are 165 665 OAs in England, each containing on average 300 people. In addition super OAs (SOAs) have been developed, which are statistical areas built from groups of OAs. There are 32 482 lower SOAs in England, each containing on average 1500 people, which combine to form 6780 middle SOAs with an average population of 7200.

Demographic segmentation is the grouping of people by other characteristics, such as age, sex, ethnicity, social class, education. This type of segmentation is very widely used to make comparisons between countries. An example is the prevalence of diabetes in men and women, which is similar until approximately age 65, when it becomes more common in women. Prevalence of diabetes is also greater in people of Asian and African origin and in indigenous peoples of the Americas and Australasia than in Caucasians.

Geo-demographic segmentation combines demographics and geography so that people are grouped within small geographic areas, but also have similar demographic characteristics. The theory is that such people are likely to have similar behaviours. The technique has been used in commercial marketing for many years, but has more recently been incorporated into public health practice in the UK. It is used to identify particular behaviours and likely responses to health messages. Several methods are available for segmenting a population into groups. An example is Mosaic public sector which segments populations into 15 groups, reflects deprivation, affluence and lifestyle and provides information at lower SOA level. Each group has been termed to illustrate the type of people within it, for example, 'new homemakers', 'active retirement' and 'elderly needs'.

Using demographic information

Demographic data can be used to highlight differences between populations, which may be due to health or other inequities. It is also used to monitor the impact of interventions. Pharmacists require a basic understanding of demographic measures so they can contribute to healthcare planning and understand the impact of their public health interventions on populations.

Geo-demographic data in particular can be used to undertake social marketing campaigns to improve the impact and effectiveness of health promotion at national and local levels. Health-related social marketing is the 'systematic application of marketing alongside other concepts and techniques to achieve specific behavioural goals to improve health and reduce inequalities'. In England, this is led by the national social marketing strategy for health.[6] An example is the marketing of public health messages about alcohol-related problems, where it is essential to first understand what type of people are at risk from high alcohol use – where they drink, what they drink and perhaps most importantly, what levers may be used to help them consider the impact of alcohol on their personal health. By identifying different kinds of drinkers, those at greatest risk can be specifically targeted, using techniques that are most likely to appeal to them and to which they can relate their behaviour.

Epidemiological data

Epidemiology is the study of the distribution and determinants of diseases or events in specific populations and the effect of interventions on these. It seeks to identify and measure factors which predispose towards, precipitate, modify, enable or reinforce a disease, condition, or disability. Studies designed to identify associations between factors and diseases and these associations can be based on populations or groups of people or on individuals.

Studies that compare populations are ecological studies. These studies compare associations between a particular illness and associated risk factors, such as lung disease and smoking. They are useful for generating ecological hypotheses about potential causes of morbidity and obtaining ecological correlations. However, in such studies, the unit of measure is the population rather than the individual, and often information from disparate groups is aggregated. Therefore any associations found apply to populations, not to individuals within those populations, because many other factors could explain differences in morbidity. Applying the findings of ecological studies to individuals leads to what is termed an 'ecological fallacy'.

There are two main types of epidemiological studies – observational and experimental. Both are most frequently conducted in individuals and thus avoid the 'ecological fallacy'.

Observational studies

Observational studies can be further divided into descriptive, in which data are gathered and presented, without evidence (inferences) made between a risk factor and the disease or event; and analytical, which seek to measure associations between potential factors which could influence the incidence or prevalence of diseases or events. These are most commonly conducted on individuals rather than on populations and can be of three types – cross sectional, case-control and cohort studies.

Cross-sectional studies

These are surveys usually conducted at a single point in time. They can collect details about demographics, disease states, symptoms, drug use, lifestyle and so on, and are often used to determine the prevalence of conditions within populations. Repeated cross-sectional surveys within the same population can be used to obtain data on how parameters change over time, providing a longitudinal dataset. They are also useful for generating hypotheses about associations between factors and diseases, however, they do not show any temporal relationship between any factor and any disease/symptom. Such hypotheses are better tested using other types of studies.

Examples of cross-section surveys are the Census, the General Household Survey (GHS, now the General Lifestyle Survey) and the Health Survey for England (HSE). They are important sources of demographic data but are widely supplemented with more local, detailed surveys. In the UK, a population census is held every 10 years, the most recent being in 2001, involving the total population. Data on sex, date of birth, ethnicity, occupation, social class, travel to work and housing tenure are usually collected. Additional data collected may vary from one census to another, so that comparisons are not always possible. In the 2001 UK Census, data were collected on the provision of unpaid care, limiting long term illness, self-reported general health and permanently sick and disabled. Most developed countries have reliable census data, but it can be less reliable in some low and middle income countries.

More detailed data are collected from a sample of households throughout the UK in the GHS which is carried out every year by the Office for National Statistics and allows estimation of the prevalence of diseases and disabilities. Data collected includes information about the people in the households, the property itself, transport, amenities, economic activity, health, disabilities and care, with descriptions of conditions experienced. Another important data source is the annual HSE, which is commissioned by the Department of Health and involves a visit to a sample of households to obtain key health outcome measures, as well as to administer a face-to-face questionnaire.

These surveys provide a wealth of information of potential value to pharmacists. For example, the 2007 GHS showed that more people in 'managerial and professional' households exceeded the daily recommended limits on their heaviest drinking day of the week than those in 'routine and manual' households, while prevalence was reversed for smoking behaviour.[7] The 2007 HSE showed that the prevalence of hypertension was 31% in men and 29% in women, of whom 46% of men and 53% of women were treated, but blood pressure was below 140/90 mmHg in 55% of those treated.[8] More women than men were aware of the recommended intake of fresh fruit and vegetables per day and of the maximum recommended units of alcohol.

Cohort studies

These are usually prospective studies (but can also be retrospective) in which a population 'cohort' of persons or patients is longitudinally monitored or followed over a long time to examine exposure to a factor of interest (or a particular characteristic). The main feature of interest is the comparison of incidence rates of a disease or an event (e.g. an adverse event, improvement in a condition, or a symptom) in subgroups that differ in exposure levels. A large population monitored over a long time period is required to generate sufficient person-years to adequately calculate differences in the incidence rates between exposures. Comparison with unexposed populations enables calculation of the degree to which exposure to the factor being studied is associated with the outcome. The results are expressed in a two-by-two table (Table 4.1).

Table 4.1

Characteristic, e.g. smoking	With outcome of interest, e.g. lung cancer	Without outcome of interest	Total
Present	a	b	a + b
Absent	c	d	c + d
Total	a + c	b + d	a + b + c + d

In cohort studies, the relative risk (RR) can be measured, because the incidence is obtainable, due to the prospective way in which such studies are carried out.

$$RR = \frac{\text{incidence rate of disease in exposed group}}{\text{incidence rate of disease in unexposed group}}$$

The incidence rate in the exposed group is calculated as $a/a+b$. That in the unexposed group is $c/c+d$. If a relative risk is less than 1, it suggests that exposure to the characteristic has a protective effect on the likelihood of developing the disease being studied. A relative risk of greater than 3.0 suggests a strong association between exposure and the disease.

For example, a cohort study of elderly people taking antidepressants found that the incidence of upper gastrointestinal (GI) bleeds in patients taking selective serotonin reuptake inhibitors (SSRIs) was 7.9/1000 person years, but 6.6/1000 person years among those taking drugs with less ability to inhibit serotonin reuptake (mainly tricyclics).

So in this case, the relative risk $= 7.9/6.6 = 1.2$, suggesting that there is a weak association between SSRIs and GI bleeds.[9]

The advantages of cohort studies are that they can be used to study multiple effects from one exposure, and they can provide measures of the incidence of the disease(s) being studied; however, they are expensive and time-consuming to conduct.

Case-control studies

Case-control studies involve two groups of patients, one of which has experienced an outcome, the other being matched in all other relevant characteristics. The patients who experienced the outcome are termed 'cases', the other group are 'controls'. The outcome may range from having a symptom or disease to an adverse effect from a drug. The purpose of the control group is to enable a comparison to be made historically about the exposure to different potential causes of the outcome being studied, such as a drug. These studies are always retrospective, because the cases have already experienced the outcome being studied. This means that they are dependent on accurate and complete records being available about exposure to the factor(s) being studied, which may be difficult to obtain.

The results from case-control studies are presented as odds ratios (ORs). As with cohort studies, they are derived from two-by-two tables as follows (Table 4.2):

Table 4.2

Characteristic, e.g. drug exposure	With event, e.g. adverse effect (cases)	Without event (controls)	Total
Present	a	b	$a + b$
Absent	c	d	$c + d$
Total	$a + c$	$b + d$	$a + b + c + d$

$$OR = \frac{a \times d}{b \times c}$$

The odds ratio explains the relative risk of the event being changed by exposure to the characteristic. Relative risk is not actually measured, because these studies are retrospective. The odds ratio approximates to relative risk. The prevalence of exposure to the characteristic among cases is calculated as $a/a + c$. That for the controls is $b/b + d$.

An example is a recent case-control study in Denmark further exploring the possible association between SSRIs and GI bleeding. The study involved 3652 cases, matched to 36 502 control patients (10 for each patient to increase the reliability of the study) and found odds ratios of 1.67, 1.88 and 1.22 for risk of upper GI bleeding in current, recent or past users of SSRIs respectively. Those taking both SSRIs and non-steroidal anti-inflammatory drugs (NSAIDs) had an odds ratio of 8.0, while those taking aspirin in addition had an odds ratio of 28.0.[10]

Case-control studies are useful because they are relatively quick and cheap to conduct, they are very good for diseases with long latency periods or rare diseases, plus multiple risk factors can also be studied at once. Because of the retrospective nature of the study, however, it can be difficult to be certain that exposure to the factor being studied did actually take place before the disease occurred, whereas in cohort studies conducted prospectively this is always true. It is also difficult to be sure other exposures which could influence outcome did not also occur, hence the importance of trying to match the case and control population for as many characteristics as possible.

Experimental studies

Experimental studies are those in which an intervention, perhaps a drug or a method of promoting healthy activity, is studied prospectively. The intervention must be compared with a control group and it is essential to ensure both populations have an equal chance of being in either group, to ensure no selection bias occurs in either the experimental or the control population, so the study used is the randomised controlled trial (RCT).

Randomised controlled trials

As with cohort studies, RCTs usually involve two groups of people or patients who are followed prospectively. The difference is that in a cohort study, which is merely observational, the investigator selects people on the basis of their existing exposure to a characteristic or factor being studied, whereas in an RCT, the investigator actually assigns the individuals to the different groups. Sometimes RCTs are not possible. For example, if you wanted to study the association between smoking and breast cancer, you could not conduct an RCT, because it is unethical to even consider allocating people randomly to smoke! You have no choice but to conduct an observational study. RCTs are experimental studies in which, as noted above, the patients included in both groups – intervention and control – should be as similar as possible in all important respects except exposure to the intervention. Randomisation helps to achieve this comparability, as do inclusion and exclusion criteria.

Pharmacists will be familiar with RCTs as a mechanism for studying the beneficial effects of drug therapy, but they can also be used for interventions that could prevent disease from developing, surgical procedures, methods of delivering services and much more.

As with cohort studies, the data from RCTs can be expressed as relative risks, because they are prospective in nature, but odds ratios are also often calculated.

In an RCT of pharmacist-led medication review, there were more pharmaceutical care issues resolved in the intervention group than in the control group.[11] Table 4.3 puts the results into a 2 × 2 table:

Table 4.3			
Intervention (medication review)	Pharmaceutical care issues resolved at follow up	Pharmaceutical care issues unresolved at follow up	Total
Present	587	256	843
Absent	136	838	974
Total	723	1094	1817

$$\text{Relative risk} = \frac{587/843}{136/974}$$

$$RR = 0.49$$

Therefore this study showed that the relative risk of having unresolved pharmaceutical care issues at follow up, if pharmacist-led medication review is provided, is around half that present if only usual care is provided.

Meta-analysis

This is the pooling of data from more than one RCT or other controlled studies in a statistically rigorous way. The main reasons for doing meta-analysis are to increase the statistical power of studies, which enables effects on subgroups to be studied and to help in making decisions about effects when there are differences in results between studies. Although the technique is regarded as the highest level of evidence, meta-analyses are dependent on the completeness of the literature review required to identify all relevant studies and on the quality of the studies included. Robust inclusion criteria are good because this ensures only the highest quality studies are included; however, it also excludes the results of many studies that are considered suboptimal. Meta-analysis can end up hiding differences between studies and must be based on trials that are sufficiently similar to allow pooling of data.

The results presented in a meta-analysis should show not only the pooled effect size, which is expressed as either relative risk or odds ratio, but also the results of the individual studies included. This is usually done in a single figure with confidence intervals being shown around the relative risk for each study in turn and a line at 1 being included, termed a Forest plot. An example is given in Figure 4.2.[12]

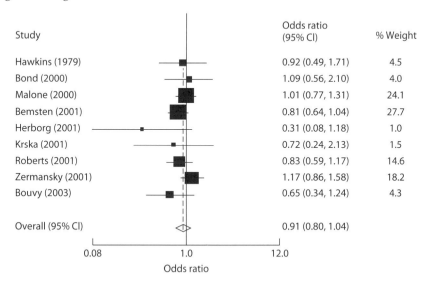

Figure 4.2   Forest plot of randomised controlled trials of pharmacist-led interventions on hospital admission.

Reproduced from Royal S, Smeaton L, Avery AJ, Hurwitz B, Sheikh A. Interventions in primary care to reduce medication-related adverse events and hospital admissions: systematic review and meta-analysis. *Qual Saf Health Care* 2006; 15: 23–31[12] with permission.

Using epidemiological data

Studying changes in the incidence and prevalence of diseases or events over time between groups of people and between geographical areas, through repeated cross-sectional surveys, can help to determine contributory factors. Studying interventions prospectively can identify the impact of these factors on the development of disease, its morbidity and mortality. Combining the results of studies undertaken in a particular area can then enable sound judgements to be made as to which factors should be avoided in the pursuit of health or whether interventions should be implemented universally to improve health.

Epidemiological studies such as surveys, cohort studies, case control studies and RCTs constitute the evidence on which national recommendations, such as those issued by NICE and SIGN, are based. Guidelines take account of the type of study and its quality by allocating a level of evidence. These are then used to assign grades of recommendation to individual guidance statements. Pharmacists may need to use these studies in their day-to-day work, whether this is in selection of drugs for formularies (see Chapter 14), guideline development, or in practising evidence-based medicine in individual patients (see Chapter 7).

Surveillance data

Public health departments throughout the world conduct ongoing health surveillance, monitoring and data analysis. Surveillance is defined as the continuous analysis, interpretation and feedback of systematically collected data. Public health surveillance provides policy makers with intelligence that allows observation of changing trends over time, place and person. This can include general or disease-specific morbidity and mortality, or characteristics which are known to influence a disease. This enables public health specialists to investigate disease outbreaks, prevent and manage epidemics and address risks to health, as well as implement public health measures to reduce the burden of disease within a population.

Surveillance systems in England

A wide variety of surveillance systems are in place in the UK, many of which are also established in other countries, particularly those for infectious diseases. Infectious diseases are particularly important to monitor to ensure control interventions are put in place for the correct population at the correct time before the disease spreads more widely. Some infectious diseases are so important that there is a statutory requirement for them to be notified to a central organisation; currently this is the Centre for

Infections of the Health Protection Agency (HPA). However, this requirement for notification of certain diseases began in the 19th century for cholera, diphtheria, smallpox and typhoid. Reporting does not require confirmation of diagnosis and the list changes as patterns of infections change. Certain hospital-acquired infections, including methicillin-resistant *Staphylococcus aureus* (MRSA) and *Clostridium difficile* are now also subject to mandatory surveillance.

For many other infectious diseases, samples of body fluids are taken and sent to laboratories for analysis. The National Laboratory Reporting Scheme gathers data from over 200 such laboratories in England and reports regularly to the HPA. These reports provide important information not only on trends and spread of infection but also on strains of causative organisms and resistance patterns.

The Royal College of General Practitioners also hosts a surveillance centre that gathers data on all patients presenting to over 100 medical practices in England and Wales every week. Weekly reports are available on a wide variety of infectious diseases, but the centre specialises in surveillance of influenza-like illness and other respiratory diseases.

The DoH gathers data from every NHS hospital in England and Wales on all admissions and day cases, stored within public health observatories. These are known as *hospital episode statistics* (HES) and contain information about dates of admission and discharge, diagnoses, treatments and operations, giving a full picture of inpatient care. Data are also gathered about diseases when patients visit GPs.

All medical practices in the UK use computer systems for patient records and appointments, many of which use one commercial system: Egton Medical Information System (EMIS). Approximately 600 of these practices now provide data on over 12 million patients for use in epidemiological studies but also provide surveillance information about infectious diseases and trends in the patterns of non-infectious diseases. Many medical practices also provide information through this system about patterns of uptake of pneumococcal and influenza vaccination.

But not everyone visits their GP when they are ill. NHS Direct is a national telephone helpline which provides information and advice to the general public on health issues at all times, through 22 call centres. All centres relay information about key symptoms reported by callers to the HPA. This provides another source of surveillance data which are used to provide early identification of epidemics or other problems.

While, at present, no such schemes involve community pharmacy, similar methods could usefully enable requests for information and advice to be collected, which could then act as markers for some public health problems, such as head lice.

Other systems and methods

In the USA, a national behavioural risk factor surveillance system is carried out by the National Center for Chronic Disease Prevention and Health Promotion, using telephone interviews. Internationally the WHO gathers data on the prevalence of disease and risk factors, to provide a global picture of health. Within England, the Association of Public Health Observatories (APHO) gathers and publishes a range of data for use by public health departments and local government. One valuable resource introduced in 2005 is the area health profile.[13] This provides information about how the health of a local population differs from the national (England) average, where inequalities are found, life expectancy in relation to deprivation, mortality trends and a range of standardised information about behaviour, hospital admissions and specific conditions.

Publications on a range of indicators of public health are also available from the APHO, such as that on drug use.[14] This document illustrates the importance of data gathering by a range of organisations which contributes to public health, not just those relating to the DoH, since it includes information from the British Crime Survey, the Offending Crime and Justice Survey, the National Drug Treatment Monitoring System and the Drug Harm Index (produced by the Home Office).

In addition to monitoring for important health conditions, surveillance must also cover issues such as environmental hazards, e.g. toxic chemicals and biological agents in the air, water, soil or in food, injuries (one of the leading causes of death and disabilities worldwide), detecting and managing outbreaks of bioterrorism, disasters, complex emergencies and refugee or homeless populations. This is to enable authorities to identify and eliminate preventable causes of illness and death in these communities.

Of course pharmacists are particularly interested in prescribing data. They need to be able to conduct epidemiological studies involving drugs – pharmacoepidemiology – and use routinely collected prescribing information to show the impact of their interventions on drug utilisation. These topics are covered in more detail in Chapter 14.

Record linkage

Record linkage, or the linking of records from different sources, sounds simple and obvious, but is actually a complex technique requiring large amounts of resource, though it has the potential to provide much more useful data for both epidemiology and surveillance. One example is the General Practice Research Database, which is the world's largest computerised database of anonymised, longitudinal, primary care medical records, managed by the Medicines and Healthcare products Regulatory Agency (MHRA).[15] The database enables diagnosis and prescribing to be linked, enabling large epidemiological studies to be conducted. In future it will also be linked to hospital records, socioeconomic data and disease registers. The database has been used to look at disease incidence, but can also be used to look at prescribing. A valuable linkage system already exists in NHS Tayside, covering primary and secondary care, which is used primarily for pharmacovigilance studies (see Chapter 14).

Using surveillance data

The generation of timely, reproducible, and accessible surveillance data facilitates the early detection of illness outbreaks and changes in disease trends over time. Continuous data gathering can also act as an early warning system for the detection of new health problems. In the case of serious and/or unexpected outbreaks of novel infectious diseases, such as severe acute respiratory syndrome (SARS) or swine flu, epidemiologists are usually sent to the area where the infection developed, to investigate the outbreak, characterise the condition and begin monitoring. An important role of these 'field epidemiologists' is to identify how diseases spread, suggest control measures and help in implementing effective recording and reporting systems. The purpose of this is to quickly contain the disease and control its spread or its impact. Naturally to achieve effective implementation of relevant health protection measures, public health departments must be responsive to the results of surveillance.

In England, the HPA is responsible for holding and updating national plans to respond to health emergencies. For example, a heatwave plan is in place, necessary because of the increased risk of high temperatures from global warming, which it is estimated could cause over 3000 immediate deaths and more than 6350 heat-related deaths throughout a single summer.[16] This has four levels of vigilance. Level 1 is 'awareness' of a potential problem, which involves the issue of general advice to public health directors and to the public, and making hospitals and primary care aware of the need to have policies ready for potential implementation in case of the situation changing to level 2. Daily reports are required by the Department of Health from this point onwards until the problem resolves, providing information on the impact and severity of temperatures on the public and how well services are responding. Level 2 is 'alert', at which point the DoH will provide specific advice to the public and advice must be distributed to at-risk individuals by primary care organisations. Level 3 is 'heatwave', during which additional care must be made available to vulnerable people and regional directors have responsibility to ensure that utilities, such as water and electricity, are not interrupted. Level 4 is 'emergency' or prolonged heatwave, which will be a major incident and all emergency policies and procedures must be applied (see Chapter 1).

An example of how this all works is given in Box 4.2.

Box 4.2 *Surveillance in England during the swine flu epidemic of 2009*

Several of the generic surveillance methods described provided continuous baseline data on the incidence of influenza. These are the National Laboratory Reporting Scheme, the RCGP weekly returns scheme and NHS Direct, together with hospital admissions caused by severe respiratory illness, and mortality monitoring from death registries.

Seasonal influenza surveillance systems were put in place as usual. These included flu as a component of data collected through medical practices.

During the build up to the epidemic, additional surveillance was put in place. This included daily case finding (organised efforts to identify as many cases as possible) through the Regional Microbiology Network and the Health Protection Agency. In addition, interviews were conducted with the first 100–200 confirmed cases, plus their contacts, to determine demographic data, symptoms, treatment and vaccination history, exposure and outcome.

Together a comprehensive picture of the progress of the epidemic was developed, enabling all staff at Primary Care Trust level to be informed daily of changes in the pattern of disease, locally, nationally and internationally. This allowed trusts to plan effectively and be prepared for the epidemic and its likely impact on the NHS and other activities.

References

1. Hill AB. The environment and disease: association or causation? *Proc Royal Soc Med* 1965; 58: 295–300.
2. Office for National Statistics. Census 2001. London: ONS, 2009. http://www.statistics.gov.uk/census2001/pyramids/pages/UK.asp.
3. Office for National Statistics Life expectancy continues to rise. London: ONS, 2009. http://www.statistics.gov.uk/cci/nugget.asp?ID=168.
4. Mathers CD, Loncar D. Projections of global mortality and burden of disease from 2002 to 2030. *PLoS Medicine* 2006; 3(11): e442.
5. Organisation for Economic Co-operation and Development Health Data, 2009. http://www.ecosante.org/index2.php?base=OCDE&langs=ENG&langh=ENG.
6. Department of Health. *Ambitions for Health: A strategic framework for maximising the potential of social marketing and health-related behaviour.* London: Department of Health, 2008. http://www.dh.gov.uk/en/Publichealth/Choosinghealth/DH_066342.
7. Office for National Statistics. *Results from the General Household Survey 2007.* London: ONS, 2008. http://www.statistics.gov.uk/StatBase/Product.asp?vlnk=5756.
8. The Information Centre, NHS. *Health Survey for England 2007.* http://www.ic.nhs.uk/pubs/hse07healthylifestyles.
9. van Walraven C, Mamdani MM, Wells PS *et al.* Inhibition of serotonin reuptake by antidepressants and upper gastrointestinal bleeding in elderly patients: retrospective cohort study. *BMJ* 2001; 323: 655–658.

10. Dall M, Ove B, Muckerdall S *et al*. An association between SSRI use and serious upper gastro-instestinal bleeding. *Clin Gastroent Hepatol* 2009; 7: 1314–1321.
11. Krska J, Cromarty JA, Arris F *et al*. Pharmacist-led medication review in patients over 65: a randomized, controlled trial in primary care. *Age Ageing* 2001; 30: 215–221.
12. Royal S, Smeaton L, Avery AJ *et al*. Interventions in primary care to reduce medication related adverse events and hospital admissions: systematic review and meta-analysis. *Qual Saf Health Care* 2006; 15: 23–31.
13. Association of Public Health Observatories. *Area Health profiles*. http://www.apho.org.uk/default.aspx?RID=49802.
14. Association of Public Health Observatories. *Indications of Public Health in English Regions. 10: Drug use*. APHO 2009. http://www.apho.org.uk/resource/item.aspx?RID=70746.
15. General Practice Research Database. http://www.gprd.com/home/default.asp.
16. Department of Health. *Heatwave plan for England 2009*. http://www.dh.gov.uk/en/publicationsandstatistics/Publications/PublicationsPolicyAndGuidance.

5

An international perspective

Ines Krass and John Bell

Public health activities of pharmacists vary in different countries depending on the prevalence of major communicable and non-communicable (chronic) diseases. This chapter includes international comparisons and provides examples of pharmacists' differing public health roles, especially in health promotion initiatives, in the developing and developed world.

Pharmacy's public health role in developing countries

Although in most high income countries the role of pharmacy in public health is widely accepted, in many developing countries the role is less well defined. In many countries there is no national health promotion strategy and community pharmacists are seen merely as shopkeepers, not health professionals. Often there is no separation between prescribing and dispensing – doctors prescribe and dispense. Conversely community pharmacists sell a wide range of medicines and are the first port of call for most of the population seeking advice and medicines. Most people in developing countries purchase all medicines themselves, rather than using government-funded sources. Other non-pharmacy outlets, such as licensed chemical sellers or drug stores, are often also permitted to sell medicines, and counterfeit medicines are often a more widespread problem than in developed countries. There is little collaboration between pharmacy, industry, government and other health professional groups. Moreover, the structure and organisation of pharmacy is not well developed and the resources of pharmacy associations are very limited.

Nevertheless pharmacists in developing countries wish to improve their status and broaden their role. They are academically highly qualified, with increasing interest and emphasis at undergraduate level on social pharmacy or pharmacy practice. In addition, governments increasingly realise that public–private partnerships can improve patient outcomes and achieve greater cost benefit. Involvement in public health initiatives can provide opportunities for individual pharmacists and the profession to be recognised as part of the healthcare team. In some countries, there are also opportunities for pharmacists to take an active role in influencing health policy and strategy by strengthening the role of professional pharmacy organisations.

In developing as well as developed countries, successful public health activities might be, and frequently are, initiated by enthusiastic individuals. However, to be effective, long term and sustainable at the population level, they must be advocated and driven by professional organisations, supported by government and ultimately expected by consumers and other stakeholders.

The variety of pharmacists' public health activities within such programmes are illustrated by examples involving both communicable and non-communicable diseases. With respect to communicable diseases we have chosen to focus on malaria, tuberculosis and HIV, since worldwide these are major causes of morbidity and mortality and public health activities targeting these conditions have been well described.

The global burden of communicable diseases

Infectious and parasitic diseases cause around 10.9 million deaths annually. Of these about 56% of deaths are caused by malaria, tuberculosis and HIV/AIDS. Thus, collectively, communicable diseases impose a huge social and economic burden on societies around the globe.[1] One of the millennium goals of the United Nations is to combat HIV/AIDS, malaria and other diseases.[2]

Malaria

Malaria is a life-threatening disease caused by parasites transmitted through bites from mosquitoes infected with the *Plasmodium* parasite. Approximately half of the world's population is at risk of contracting malaria; however, those living in tropical regions of low and middle income countries are most vulnerable. Although preventable and curable, 247 million cases of malaria were recorded in 2006, causing nearly one million deaths, mostly among children under five years in sub-Saharan Africa.[3]

Local factors, such as rainfall patterns (mosquitoes breed in wet conditions), the proximity to people of mosquito breeding sites such as stagnant water and types of mosquito species, affect malaria transmission rates. While, some regions are 'malaria endemic' with a constant number of cases, other areas have 'malaria seasons' usually coinciding with the rainy season. Malaria imposes a significant economic burden in high-rate areas, disproportionately affects poor people who cannot afford treatment or have limited access to healthcare and traps families and communities in a downward poverty spiral.[3]

Early treatment of malaria shortens its duration and prevents complications plus most deaths. Artemisinin-based combination therapies are the best available treatment. However, increasingly drug resistance is undermining malaria control efforts. There are no effective alternatives for malaria treatment on the market or in late stages of development, so prevention is key to malaria control. Prevention focuses on reducing disease transmission by controlling the malaria-bearing mosquito through the use of insecticide-treated nets for night-time prevention of bites and indoor residual spraying to kill mosquitoes resting on house walls and roofs. Resistance to insecticides, however, is also a growing problem.

Pharmacists' activities in malaria: Zimbabwe, Ghana and Tanzania

In 2001 the Pharmaceutical Society of Zimbabwe, with the support of the Commonwealth Pharmacists Association, produced and distributed a consumer-focused malaria fact card (MFC). This aimed to increase community awareness of malaria prevention and treatment in the community and reinforce the need for early diagnosis and treatment. It also provided a basis for training pharmacists and their staff in best practice guidelines for prevention and locally relevant malaria treatment. The template for the programme was the highly successful Pharmacy Self Care programme developed in Australia in the 1980s. The Australian programme, supported by government and industry, promotes pharmacy's professional role and provides up-to-date, authoritative and objective health information to the consumer. It includes 80 consumer-oriented fact cards (revised annually) in 14 categories.

The MFC required collaborative development between the Zimbabwean pharmaceutical society and the departments of pharmaceutical services and epidemiology and disease control within the Ministry of Health. Local industry and the Retail Pharmacists Association sponsored the printing and assisted with the distribution of the cards. Initially produced in English and distributed to three urban centres, the card was subsequently distributed more widely and translated into two local languages (Figure 5.1). It provided a mechanism for publicising changes to health ministry treatment guidelines in 2003.

In Ghana, their pharmaceutical society recognised the need to ensure that both community pharmacies and licensed chemical sellers provided accurate and up-to-date consumer advice to complement the government's information, education and communication strategy to increase community awareness of malaria prevention, transmission and treatment. The society trained large numbers of pharmacists to use the MFC as a consumer counselling tool. Launched during Malaria Awareness Week in 2002 using a national television presentation, the cards were distributed to pharmacies, licensed

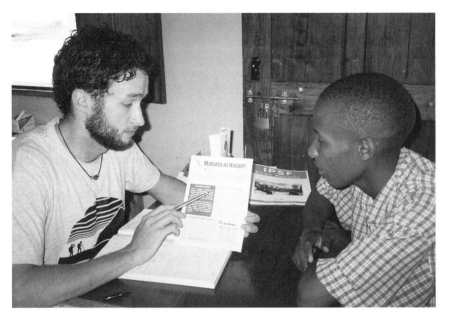

Figure 5.1   Malaria fact card in action.

chemical sellers and clinics throughout Ghana and by 2004 it had been translated from the original English into six local languages. Pharmacists subsequently became trainers of non-pharmacy healthcare workers to ensure competence in discussing the card with consumers. Evaluation of the society's intervention by consumer surveys showed that over 70% of consumers obtained previously unknown information about prevention and treatment and intended to take the card home to inform family and friends.

The important issues identified by the Pharmaceutical Society of Tanzania were lack of knowledge about transmission, delay in seeking healthcare and minimal resources to purchase medications. These were major contributors to high rates of malaria among low income urban dwellers in Dar-es-Salaam. MFCs were printed in Swahili, endorsed by the national malaria control programme and launched by the Tanzanian prime minister in 2002 during the change in national treatment guidelines. The MFC provided advice on personal protection strategies, early symptoms, especially in children, and information on how to take antimalarial medication. Evaluation of the society's intervention showed that just over 74% of consumers increased their knowledge of antimalarial treatment including method of administration and possible side effects.

Tuberculosis

Tuberculosis is transmitted by airborne spread of the bacterium, *Mycobacterium tuberculosis*. When infected people cough, sneeze, talk or spit, they propel tuberculosis bacilli into the air, and inhaling only a small number causes infection. If untreated, each person with active disease will infect on average between 10 and 15 people every year. However, people infected with tuberculosis bacilli will not necessarily develop active disease. The immune system isolates the bacilli, which, protected by a thick waxy coat, can lie dormant for years. Typically, infection is confined to the lungs but it may also affect bones, blood and other body organs. Although a third of the world's population is currently infected with the bacillus, only 5–10% of people become sick or infectious at some time during their life. People infected with HIV, however, are much more likely to develop tuberculosis. Globally, the burden of tuberculosis is increasing due to poverty in various populations, e.g. developing countries, disadvantaged urban populations in developed countries, inadequate case detection, diagnosis and treatment, drug resistance, poor health infrastructure and the impact of the HIV pandemic.[4]

According to WHO estimates published in 2009, the largest number of new tuberculosis cases occurred in South-East Asia, accounting for 34% of global incidence. However, the estimated incidence in sub-Saharan Africa is nearly twice that of South-East Asia, at nearly 350 cases per 100 000 population per year. Figure 5.2 compares the prevalence of tuberculosis in selected countries in Europe, Australasia, Asia and Africa.[5]

The highest number of deaths and the highest mortality per capita both occur in Africa and a third of these occur in HIV-positive individuals. The

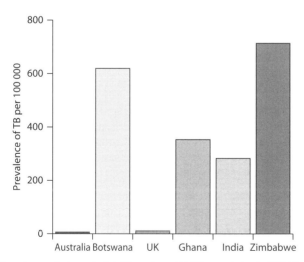

Figure 5.2 Prevalence of tuberculosis (all forms) per 100 000 population in 2007. Reproduced with permission from WHO.

tuberculosis epidemic in Africa grew rapidly during the 1990s, but the incidence has now stabilised and begun decreasing. However, this is offset by population growth, consequently, the number of new cases arising each year is still increasing globally especially in Africa, the Eastern Mediterranean and South-East Asia.[5]

The main intervention for tuberculosis control is a standardised course of combination chemotherapy. In the initial two-month treatment phase, the regimen should include at least four drugs and be supervised, i.e. given as directly observed treatment, short-course (DOTS). In the four-month continuation phase, at least three of the most active and best-tolerated drugs should be given. Combining agents reduces the likelihood of drug resistance, which can be a major barrier to treatment success. Poor adherence to or premature interruption of treatment however, undermines this benefit[4] and is a frequent occurrence, representing a further significant barrier to disease control.

In patients with HIV-related tuberculosis, the priority is to treat tuberculosis, especially smear-positive pulmonary cases. However, with careful management, these patients can receive concomitant antiretroviral therapy.

Pharmacists' activities in tuberculosis: India

India bears the greatest burden of tuberculosis globally, accounting for a fifth of cases worldwide. The government of India, through the Revised National Tuberculosis Control Programme,[6] has rapidly expanded treatment services and is collaborating with private sector providers to research models that promote equitable and sustainable provision of treatment within internationally recognised standards and guidelines. Despite free treatment being available at government centres, up to 80% of people in India seek it from private sector physicians, pharmacists and traditional medicine providers. This is reportedly because of the cost of travel to government clinics, long waiting times, limited hours of opening, poor service and stigma associated with attending such clinics.

Within this context the Indian Pharmaceutical Association, the Commonwealth Pharmacists Association and the International Pharmaceutical Students' Federation collaborated on a pilot project in Mumbai assessing the preparedness of community pharmacies to undertake training to provide DOTS.[6] An information, education and communication strategy was developed to raise community awareness of tuberculosis for delivery through community pharmacies, including a fact card. After training, pharmacists used the card to counsel patients on use of their medications during DOTS, since high quality patient/pharmacist interaction has been shown to aid adherence to long term therapy. Selected community pharmacists in Mumbai have since been registered with the programme as treatment providers, giving patients alternative local options for convenient and confidential DOTS.

HIV/AIDS

HIV is a retroviral infection, which first appeared approximately 30 years ago. Since the first cases were indentified in the United States, it has escalated into a devastating global epidemic resulting in approximately 25 million deaths.[7] It is transmitted through both heterosexual and homosexual contact, from mother to fetus or baby, blood transfusion and contact with contaminated blood products, e.g., shared needles by injecting drug users. Globally, heterosexual transmission is the most common route of infection, especially in developing countries. In the initial phase, HIV attacks CD4+ helper T-lymphocytes and causes an intense viraemia when the infected cells enter the circulation. The acute illness is usually self limited, once the host's immune response brings the infection under relative control. However, control is never complete and viral replication continues, resulting in progressive depletion of CD4+ helper T-lymphocytes over time. The rate of disease progression depends on the viral load, which in turn may be influenced by a number of host factors, including concomitant infections. Advanced disease or AIDS (autoimmune deficiency syndrome) is characterised by severely compromised immunity leading to opportunistic infections such as disseminated cytomegalovirus, mucosal candidiasis, pneumoncystis pneumonia and Kaposi's sarcoma.[7]

Globally an estimated 33 million people live with HIV/AIDS.[7] Sub-Saharan Africa bears the major burden of disease, accounting for 67% of all people living with HIV/AIDS and 75% of AIDS deaths in 2007 (Figure 5.3). In countries such as Botswana, South Africa and Zimbabwe, infection among expectant mothers is consistently over 20%.[8] In virtually all regions outside of sub-Saharan Africa, AIDS disproportionately affects injecting drug users, men who have sex with men and sex workers.[7]

While HIV/AIDS was once a rapidly fatal disease, the advent of highly active antiretroviral therapy has dramatically improved survival. Nowadays, many AIDS patients have to contend with other challenges. These include the

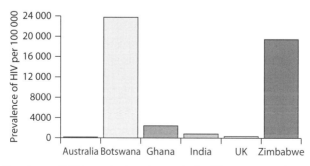

Figure 5.3 Prevalence of HIV in a selection of countries in different regions. Reproduced with permission from WHO.

non-infectious complications of their disease, e.g. AIDS-related malignancies, chronic renal failure and the long term adverse effects of antiretroviral therapy (e.g. lipodystrophy, insulin resistance, cardiovascular disease and osteoporosis).

Notwithstanding the availability of effective therapy, the global epidemic persists. Although access to treatments in the developing world has improved over time as a result of a number of key global initiatives, they are not available to all populations.[9] Other serious obstacles in the fight against HIV/AIDS relate to social stigma and discrimination against people living with HIV/AIDS, persistence of behaviours that facilitate transmission (notably unsafe sexual practice and needle sharing) and the socioeconomic barriers such as homophobia and the low status of women in many societies. These can preclude access to treatment and support services.[9] (See Figure 5.4.)

Prevention, especially by way of safe-sex practices, also has a pivotal role to play in containing the epidemic. Implementation of universal HIV testing, early provision of antiretroviral therapy to prevent AIDS, opioid substitution programmes and the provision of clean needles for drug users have all been important and successful interventions for HIV prevention. However, prevention programmes have not always been adequately resourced or appropriately targeted to the most vulnerable groups.[9]

Pharmacists' activities in HIV/AIDS: Kenya, Nigeria and Australia

In Kenya, the *Nairobi Statement on the Role of the Pharmacist in the Prevention and Management of HIV/AIDS in Kenya*[10] was developed through facilitated workshops held on World AIDS Day, 2006. This workshop, hosted by the Pharmaceutical Society of Kenya and the Commonwealth Pharmacists Association, brought together major stakeholders in HIV/AIDS prevention and management and enabled pharmacists to engage with government to identify new ways to proactively address the urgent need to reduce HIV transmission and improve access to treatment. Recommendations included:

- the use of voluntary rotations of pharmacists, in both public and private sectors and in rural and remote areas
- pharmacists' use of the media in AIDS education programmes
- an expanded role for pharmacists in the treatment of opportunistic infections
- improved supportive care of patients, especially in the area of nutrition
- encouragement of pharmacists to take a greater role in community/family/ workplace information and awareness activities.

The Live Well Initiative (LWI)[11] is a pharmacist-developed and pharmacist-led public health, non-government organisation based in Nigeria. The LWI mission is to 'improve health status through wellness promotion and health empowerment and thereby positively influencing health-seeking behaviour'.

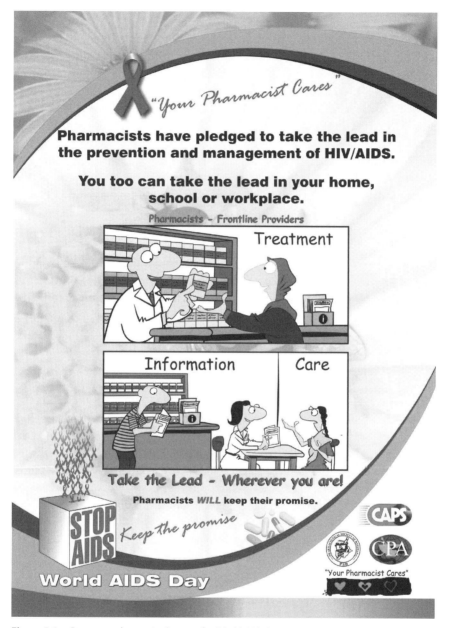

Figure 5.4 Botswana pharmacists' poster for World Aids Day.

One of LWI's activities is the HIV/AIDS enlightenment programme, which focuses on advocacy through the 'abc' concept of HIV/AIDS prevention:

- *a*bstinence
- *b*eing faithful
- *c*ondom use.

In its HIV/AIDS prevention outreach programmes, LWI pharmacists, doctors and nurses work collaboratively to target young people, vulnerable adults and highly mobile populations such as long distance truck drivers. LWI designs and delivers training for pharmacists and other health professionals in HIV/AIDS prevention, testing, counselling and treatment.

In many developed countries, including Australia, the provision of clean needles to injecting drug users has been a key, if sometimes controversial, strategy to minimise the transmission of HIV. Australia's needle and syringe programmes (NSPs) have been one of the most successful public health initiatives over the last 20 years,[12] since drug users there are one of the few injecting drug-using communities in the world who have avoided a major HIV epidemic. Through NSPs, pharmacists play a pivotal role in preventing the spread of other blood-borne viruses such as hepatitis B and hepatitis C (see Chapter 12).

Involvement in NSPs is voluntary, with approximately 50% of community pharmacies nationwide participating in the programmes. Funding is provided centrally by government and programmes are administered by the various states. In New South Wales (NSW) about half the total NSP outlets are in pharmacies (435) and pharmacies in NSW distribute over two million syringes each year. Clients can either exchange packs of (usually five) syringes at no cost or buy packs of clean syringes. The pharmacies accept returns of used needles for safe disposal and are paid by the NSW Health Department for each pack returned.

Another widespread approach to reducing injecting drug use is the opioid substitution programme.[13] In NSW for example, over 500 pharmacies provide dosing services to more than 7000 patients on a daily basis. An incentive scheme operates to encourage pharmacists to dispense methadone or buprenorphine as part of their mainstream services. Medicines are provided to the pharmacist by the government at no cost and the patients are charged for the service. This is in contrast to systems in the UK, where supervision of methadone consumption is an enhanced, locally commissioned pharmacy service, but one that is free to patients.

The global burden of chronic diseases

The main life-threatening chronic diseases worldwide include cardiovascular diseases, mainly heart disease and stroke, cancer, chronic respiratory diseases and diabetes. A common set of modifiable risk factors interacting with age and heredity, explain the alarming increase in prevalence of these conditions (see Chapter 2). Notably, the relationship between the major modifiable risk factors and the main chronic diseases is similar in all regions of the world. The spiralling epidemics of chronic disease occurring internationally, however, are also the product of societal structures which strongly influence individual health behaviour (see Chapter 2).[14] In other words being poor, unemployed and disempowered in either a developed or developing country increases the risk of engaging in unhealthy behaviours such as smoking and poor diet and also of experiencing mental health problems. A growing body of research suggests that inequalities within societies have an equal or greater impact on the overall health of the society than income disparities between countries.[15]

In 2005, chronic diseases took the lives of over 35 million people world-wide, including many young people and those in middle age. In the US alone, the total impact of these diseases on the economy is $1.3 trillion annually. Of this amount, lost productivity totals $1.1 trillion per year, while another $277 billion is spent annually on treatment.[16] Over time with increases in life expectancy and falling birth rates, chronic diseases have now overtaken communicable diseases as the main causes of death in most regions of the world. The total number of people dying from chronic diseases is double that of all infectious diseases, maternal and prenatal conditions and nutritional deficiencies combined in all regions except Africa (Figure 5.5). This is inevitable in the short term when premature deaths from infectious diseases fall (secondary to the introduction of programmes to reduce infectious disease mortality), until effective preventative measures for chronic disease are introduced and taken up.

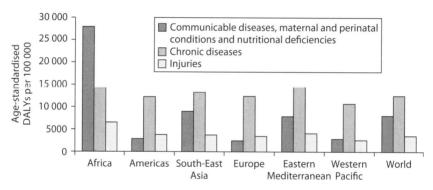

Figure 5.5 Projected main causes of the burden of disease in males (DALYs by WHO region), all ages, 2005. From http://www.who.int/chp/chronic_disease_report/part2_ch1/en/index7.html Reproduced with permission from WHO.

In the early decades of the 20th century, heart disease was common only in high income countries; however, the epidemic has now spread globally to middle and low income countries. Diabetes and obesity are also increasing at an exponential rate in all regions of the world. Alarmingly, 80% of chronic disease deaths now occur in low and middle income countries and half are in women. Without action to address the causes, deaths from chronic diseases will increase by 17% between 2005 and 2015.[17]

Pharmacist activities in non-communicable diseases: Cameroon, Fiji and Brazil

The World Diabetes Foundation states that sustainable care in developing countries depends on increasing awareness of diabetes, prevention of diabetes and its complications, education and training of patients and healthcare professionals and enhancing the detection, treatment and monitoring of diabetes. Pharmacists' traditional involvement in medication management for people with diabetes has extended to screening services in a number of countries. Most successful initiatives involve partnerships with other health professionals and national or local organisations.

In many developing countries where communicable diseases such as HIV/AIDS, tuberculosis and malaria remain the more visible and immediate threat to health, educating communities about diabetes is essential in preventing and managing the condition. In the context of traditional sociocultural beliefs and practices, raising awareness of the early signs and symptoms of diabetes and accessing treatment, presents public health professionals with significant challenges. Inadequate healthcare infrastructure and limited resources for implementing and promoting diabetes services also remain major constraints in stemming the increasing prevalence of diabetes and other chronic diseases.

On World Diabetes Day 2007,[18] the first such day recognised by the United Nations, pharmacists raised awareness of the early warning signs of diabetes and promoted healthy lifestyles in a pan-Commonwealth effort to help prevent type 2 diabetes in children, using the banner 'Your pharmacist cares about you, your child and diabetes'. Pharmacies in Cameroon conducted foot health checks. Pharmacies in Fiji provided blood glucose and blood pressure monitoring, calculated body mass indexes and advised patients on optimal weight range, diet and physical activity.[19]

In Brazil, a four-year 'diabetes treatment and resource mobilisation' project was launched in March 2006 with the aim of improving diabetes treatment in 51 low income, medium size cities.[20] Pharmacists and other health professionals work with the National Federation of Diabetes Associations and Entities in train-the-trainer programmes specifically to improve prevention of diabetes-related blindness. Events associated with World Diabetes Day in Brazil have included screening camps to detect diabetes and associated complications in people with limited access to healthcare clinics and diabetes services. Pharmacists and other health professionals volunteering their services at the Sao Paulo camp in 2007 screened more than 11 000 people over a three-day period.

International opportunities for pharmacists

There are many opportunities for pharmacists trained in developed countries to work in developing countries where public health principles underlie the majority of pharmacy-related activities in the community. To do so, an understanding of both local issues and global and national medicines policies is essential. Pharmacists working in volunteer or consultant positions with international non-governmental organisations are generally involved with policy development (including national treatment guidelines), drug selection and distribution and development and delivery of education and training programs.

International Pharmaceutical Students' Federation

The International Pharmaceutical Students' Federation (IPSF) has a particular focus on public health, with specific programmes on counterfeit medicines, diabetes, HIV/AIDS, tuberculosis and tobacco control. Internships with the Stop Tuberculosis Partnership and the Department of Chronic Diseases and Health Promotion at WHO are occasionally available through IPSF.[21] The Neema village project administered by IPSF was established in 1993 with the goal of setting up a dispensary and healthcare clinic in a remote area of Tanzania, staffed during the first three years by a rotation of international pharmacy students and Tanzanian health professionals. The centre was officially opened in 2001 and handed over to the Tanzanian government in 2004.

Currently IPSF is coordinating the Mobile Pharmacy in Northern Uganda Project[22] to assist in providing healthcare to people living in refugee camps around Gulu. As with the Neema project, two or three pharmacy students on three to six month rotations will help staff the clinic.

Fédération Internationale Pharmaceutique

The Fédération Internationale Pharmaceutique (FIP) provides opportunities for pharmacists with an interest in public health to collaborate with like-minded colleagues. Public health projects, recently completed or now being undertaken, include patient safety, counterfeit medicines, HIV/AIDS, malaria and Pharmacists and Action on Tobacco.[23]

Voluntary Service Overseas

Voluntary Service Overseas (VSO) is an international federation of member organisations that all contribute resources to a shared development programme which aims to aims to tackle poverty by using the skills, commitment and enthusiasm of individuals from around the world. Their members are based in Canada, Kenya, the Netherlands, the Philippines and the UK. They partner with Australian Volunteers International in Australia and they also recruit volunteers in India through iVolunteer. VSO also recruits and raises funds in the UK and Ireland. The organisation recruits volunteers aged between 18 and 75 to live and work in the heart of local communities. Pharmacists can volunteer to serve abroad and if they are or have been employees of the NHS in Britain, the NHS will support them to work for VSO by, for example, continuing their pension contributions while they are away.[24]

In conclusion, there is enormous scope for pharmacists to contribute to public health efforts internationally. With the ongoing burden of communicable diseases and the rising prevalence of non-communicable lifestyle diseases, such as diabetes and cardiovascular disease, there is an urgent need to mobilise all available resources in the healthcare sector. By proactively engaging in health promotion and prevention programmes, pharmacists can strengthen their position as key players in the healthcare team. Although there is mounting evidence that pharmacists already play a constructive and valuable role, there is much room to expand their participation in public health in all countries.

References

1. World Health Organization. *World Health Report, 2004.* http://whqlibdoc.who.int/whr/2004/924156265X.pdf (accessed 16 September, 2009).
2. World Health Organization. *Health and Millenium Development Goals, 2000.* http://www.who.int/mdg/mdg_poster.pdf (accessed 16 September, 2009).
3. World Health Organization. *World Malaria Report, 2008.* http://apps.who.int/malaria/wmr2008/ (accessed 7 September, 2009).
4. World Health Organization. *Treatment Of Tuberculosis: Guidelines for national programmes 3rd edition. 2003* [updated 9th September, 2009]. http://whqlibdoc.who.int/hq/2003/WHO_CDS_TB_2003.313_eng.pdf
5. World Health Organization. *WHO Report 2009 – Global tuberculosis control 2009.* http://www.who.int/tb/publications/global_report/2009/key_points/en/index.html (accessed 7 September 2009).
6. TBC India. *Revised National Tuberculosis Control Plan (RNTCP).* 2006. http://www.tbcindia.org/RNTCP.asp (accessed 6 October, 2009).
7. UNAIDS. *2008 report on the Global AIDS epidemic.* 2008. http://www.unaids.org/en/KnowledgeCentre/HIVData/GlobalReport/2008/2008_Global_report.asp (accessed 2 September, 2009).
8. Sharma SK, Kadhiravan T. Management of the patient with HIV disease. *Dis Mon* 2008; 54: 162–195.
9. Piot P, Kazatchkine M, Dybul M *et al*. AIDS: lessons learnt and myths dispelled. *Lancet* 2009; 374: 260–263.
10. Commonwealth Pharmacists Association. *The Nairobi Statement On The Role of the Pharmacist in the Prevention & Management of HIV/AIDS in Kenya.* 2006. http://www.commonwealthpharmacy.org/resources/downloads/pdfs/Nairobi_Statement.pdf (accessed 6 October 2009].
11. The LiveWell Initiative (LWI). http://www.livewellng.org/home.html (accessed 6 October 2009).
12. Law MG, Batey RG. Injecting drug use in Australia: needle/syringe programs prove their worth, but hepatitis C still on the increase. *Med J Aust* 2003; 178: 197–198.
13. The Pharmacy Guild of Australia NSW. *Dependency Care.* 2009. http://www.guild.org.au/nsw/content.asp?id=1080 (accessed 14 October 2009).
14. Marmot M. Social determinants of health inequalities. *Lancet* 2005; 365: 1099–104.
15. Wilkinson R, Pickett K. *The Spirit Level: Why equality is better for everyone.* London: Penguin Books, 2009.

16. DeVol R, Bedroussian A, Charuworn A *et al. An Unhealthy America: The economic burden of chronic disease – charting a new course to save lives and increase productivity and economic growth.* 2007. http://www.milkeninstitute.org/publications/publications.taf?function=detail&ID=38801018&cat=ResRep (accessed 21 September 2009).

17. World Health Organization. *Chronic Diseases and Health Promotion 2009.* http://www.who.int/chp/chronic_disease_report/part2_ch1/en/index1.html (accessed 13 September 2009).

18. World Diabetes Day. 2007–8. http://www.worlddiabetesday.org/en/the-campaign/previous-campaigns/2007–2008 (accessed 14th October 2009).

19. Commonwealth Pharmaceutical Association Annual Health Awareness Campaign 2007–2008 'Your Pharmacist Cares' World Diabetes Day – 14 November 2007. http://www.commonwealthpharmacy.org/resources/downloads/pdfs/World_Diabetes_Day_2007.pdf (accessed 15 October 2009).

20. World Diabetes Foundation. *Diabetes Treatment and Resource Mobilization 2006.* http://www.worlddiabetesfoundation.org/composite-939.htm (accessed 15 October 2009).

21. International Pharmaceutical Students' Federation. *Public Health Partnerships.* 2009. http://www.ipsf.org/internships.php (accessed 6 October 2009).

22. International Pharmaceutical Students' Federation. *ISPF Newsletter.* 2009. http://www.ipsf.org/userfiles/File/Newsletter%2064.pdf (accessed 6 October 2009).

23. International Pharmaceutical Federation. *FIP Programmes and Projects.* 2009. http://www.fip.org/www/?page=projects_and_programmes (accessed 6 October 2009).

24. VSO United Kingdom. 2010 [cited 29 May 2010]; http://www.vso.org.uk/

SECTION 2

Developing pharmacy public health services

6

Needs assessment and public involvement

Fiona Harris

Health needs assessment

This chapter gives an overview of what a health needs assessment (HNA) is, why it is needed and how it is used, and to explain why it is increasingly important to pharmacists and pharmaceutical services. HNA is a systematic method of identifying the health needs, with or without social care, of a population. Based on the assessments, recommendations for specific services are made. The overall aim of an HNA is to provide information to the organisations that are responsible for planning and ensuring delivery of health and social care services, to help them improve the health of the population for whom they are responsible.[1] Within the NHS this is usually primary care organisations such as a PCT in England or a health board in Scotland, Wales and Northern Ireland. However, HNAs can involve anything that impacts on health, including services within the remit of local government, as these can affect the wider determinants of health. They can be carried out for large populations (such as that covered by a PCT) and smaller populations (such as those served by an individual medical practice or community pharmacy).

Although the term HNA was only introduced in the early 1990s, the principles of assessing the needs of a population have been around for a long time. In the 19th century the first medical officers for health were responsible for assessing the needs of their local populations.[2] In the 1970s fair distribution of resources within the NHS required the assessment of relative health needs on the basis of standard mortality ratios and socioeconomic deprivation. The 1992 *Health of the Nation* initiative was a government attempt to assess national health needs and to determine priorities for improving health.[3]

HNA is now considered to be an objective and valid method of tailoring health services to the specific needs of a population. In essence it is an evidence-based approach to commissioning and planning health and social care services. Although traditionally HNAs have been undertaken by public health specialists within commissioning or purchasing organisations, as the NHS moves towards a more preventive model, all health professionals must understand local health needs. Anyone who is involved in developing services should do so in accordance with the needs of their local population. Combining population needs assessment with personal knowledge of patients' needs may help to achieve this.[4]

Why is health needs assessment important?

In recent years medical care has advanced and improved, while there have been significant changes in demography within the UK and elsewhere. These changes have led to an increase in the demand for and cost of health services, so much so that healthcare is now one of the largest sectors in most developed countries. There has also been a rise in expectations, not only in what services are available and to whom (access and equity) but also in the quality of those services (appropriateness and effectiveness).

However, the resources available for healthcare are finite, and very few, if any, governments are able to provide such care universally. Therefore access to healthcare can be inequitable, not only in terms of the people who can and do access services but also where and when services are provided. Availability of services has been shown to be inversely related to the need of the population served.[5]

Conducting a health needs assessment

Before starting any HNA, it is first essential to understand what is meant by the need for health and for healthcare.

Defining need, supply and demand

Need is an interesting concept and much has been written on the subject.[6,7] Healthcare professionals, sociologists, philosophers, and economists all have different views of what needs are.[2] But 'need', or more specifically 'health need', must be differentiated from demand and supply. In the context of HNA 'need' is usually used in relation to healthcare, i.e. the need for healthcare, which is very different from the need for health. The latter is much wider in definition, incorporating the wider social and economic determinants of health. Health needs of a population will be constantly changing and many of the wider health needs are not amenable to medical intervention.[1,2]

In healthcare, need is commonly defined as 'capacity to benefit'. In essence if healthcare needs are to be identified then an effective intervention should be available to meet these needs and the result should be an improvement in health. Where there is no effective intervention or no resources available to fund an intervention, there will be no benefit (this may be the identification of health need rather than healthcare need). If there is no benefit for whatever reason, it is often described as 'unmet need'.

Demand, on the other hand, is what people ask for or are willing to pay for, and can be influenced by a variety of factors including individual knowledge, attitudes/beliefs, media interest or availability. Demand can also be influenced by supply, for instance pharmaceutical products often create demand because they are available rather than there is a specific need. An example would be antibiotics given for a viral infection.

Supply is what is actually provided. Supply depends on the interests of health professionals, the priorities of politicians, and the amount of money/resource available. Variation in these factors frequently leads to geographical differences in supply.[1,2] However, need, demand, and supply overlap, and this relationship is important to consider when assessing health needs (Figure 6.1).

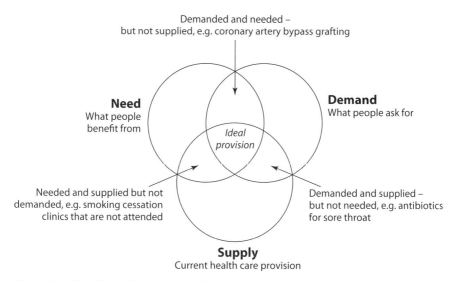

Figure 6.1 The relationship between need, demand and supply. Adapted from Stevens A, Gabbay J. Needs Assessment, needs assessment. *Health Trends* 1991; 23: 20–23 with permission.[8]

Approaches to health needs assessment

A number of approaches to conducting HNAs have been suggested[1]:

- *epidemiological:* based on prevalence and/or incidence of condition combined with clinical and cost-effectiveness of potential interventions where appropriate

- *comparative:* based on comparisons between local services and those elsewhere
- *corporate:* based on views of interested parties (for example, patients, healthcare professionals and local politicians).

To be able to examine 'capacity to benefit', HNAs must incorporate assessments of clinical effectiveness and cost-effectiveness together with patients' perspectives. This enables the balancing of clinical, ethical and economic considerations of need, i.e. what should be done, what can be done, and what can be afforded. However, it is also worth recognising that the 'capacity [of a population] to benefit' is often greater than the available resources and therefore assessments should also incorporate questions about setting priorities.[9]

Generally an HNA provides the opportunity for[2]:

- describing the patterns of disease in the local population and how these may differ from health or local authority, regional, or national disease patterns
- learning more about the needs and priorities of the local population
- highlighting the areas of unmet need and providing a clear set of objectives to meet them
- deciding rationally how to use resources to improve the local population's health in the most effective and efficient way
- influencing policy, multi-agency/partnership working, or research and development priorities.

Importantly, HNAs also provide a method of monitoring and promoting equity in the provision and use of health services and addressing inequalities in health.[2]

The importance of assessing health needs rather than reacting to health demands is widely recognised but there is no easy template for undertaking an assessment. Each will require a different approach depending on the questions being asked but will usually involve a combination of qualitative and quantitative information, together with adapting and transferring what is already known or available. A list of useful questions is provided in Table 6.1 (adapted from references 1 and 2), to form a starting point for an HNA.

Gathering information for health needs assessment

Data and information for an HNA can be obtained from a variety of different sources. Some are nationally available such as census and mortality data, hospital usage data and evaluation of interventions such as NICE appraisals. Some may be available locally, such as information on use and costs of local services. It may also be necessary to undertake local

Table 6.1 Questions to be answered by a health needs assessment	
Question	**Work required to answer it**
What is the problem?	Identify the problem to be addressed in a defined population
	Broad: e.g. people with learning disabilities, ethnic minorities, elderly people
	Focused: e.g. people with stroke, epilepsy or diabetes, people living in a particular deprived area
What is the size and nature of the problem?	Identify how many people in the defined population are likely to have the target condition or conditions, what their characteristics are, to what extent are they already receiving effective interventions, and will they be able to access new services effectively
What are the current services?	Identify what treatments or interventions are currently available to the population and how effective they are in terms of outcomes
What do patients/users want?	Identify the views of local stakeholders:
	Patients/users, carers, healthcare professionals, local politicians, voluntary groups and the local community
	Use interviews, questionnaires, focus groups and health panels/events
What are the most appropriate, cost-effective and clinically effective solutions?	Identify potentially clinically and cost-effective interventions by searching the literature and determine effectiveness through national evaluations (NICE) or local evaluations/audit
What are the resource implications?	Identify the costs of competing interventions in the context of the outcomes each is likely to achieve. Identify the risks of not meeting the need
What outcomes will demonstrate change and what criteria are needed to audit practice?	Identify what needs to be monitored/measured to show that the health benefits predicted actually occur
Adapted from references 1 and 2.	

data gathering. This may involve quantitative data from surveys of defined populations, designed to answer specific questions and qualitative data obtained through local consultations to understand what patients want.

There is a wealth of data available within the NHS but not all of it is useful information and, in common with many other organisations, the NHS spends a lot of time collecting it. Unfortunately, 'Murphy's law of information' plays a part at this stage: 'The information we have is not what we want. The information we want is not what we need'. However, routinely available data can be used, even if this entails some compromise in terms of precision. Used with survey information, routinely collected data can provide a powerful assessment of health needs and use of services. Therefore it is important to concentrate on gathering the information that will give the most useful insights (that is, answer the questions being asked as far as possible) rather than collecting all sorts of data that might turn out not to be relevant.[10] It should also be remembered that none of the routinely available data is without some form of error or bias therefore any HNA should consider the information in light of these potential errors and discuss the implications for the assessment. Some useful sources of health information available in England are shown in Box 6.1 (see also Chapter 4). Similar sources are available in many other countries. In addition, insurance companies can be an important source in countries with healthcare systems based largely on insurance.

Involving patients and the public

Patients often have a different perception of what would make them healthier: a job, a bus route to the hospital, or some advice on benefits, for example. It is increasingly important to obtain input from patients and the public to gain a 'consumer perspective' of need. However, beyond the requirement to gain patient and public input to support HNAs, public organisations such as the NHS and local government are accountable to the public and therefore have a responsibility to gain their input into how services are planned, commissioned and delivered.[12] Indeed, strategic health authorities, PCTs and acute NHS trusts must by law make arrangements for people who receive or may receive services to be involved in service planning, proposals for changing services and any decision making that affects services. In addition, one of the key objectives of the Next Stage Review of the NHS, commissioned by the DoH in 2008,[13] is that patients and the public should be empowered, giving them more rights and control over their own health and care.

Local involvement networks (LINks) have been established throughout the country, which are groups of local people and bodies set up to ensure that local communities can monitor service provision, influence key decisions and have a stronger voice in the process of commissioning health and social care. LINks are an important source of local opinion that assist PCTs in determining the health and social care needs of local people.[14] There are many other ways of involving the public in identifying needs (Box 6.2).

However, gaining the view of some groups of people, such as those with learning disabilities is not straightforward and another approach is required. Advocacy involves drawing attention to problems, speaking up for the local community and influencing policies to effect change and is an important element of promoting health and well-being. Advocacy can be carried out

Box 6.1 *National sources of health information in England, based on reference 11*

Population

- Census data can be used to describe populations at a district or electoral ward level by age, sex, ethnic group or socioeconomic status (www.statistics.gov.uk).
- Census information along with other national information sources on variables such as unemployment, overcrowding, access to services, educational achievement is used to produce indices of deprivation for super output areas (www.communities.gov.uk).

Mortality

- National registration of deaths and causes of death provide comprehensive (though not always accurate) information on mortality (www.nchod.org.uk).
- Perinatal and infant mortality 'rates' (they are not rates but proportions) are used for comparisons of the quality of healthcare.
- Standardised mortality ratios are used to compare local information on total mortality or mortality from specific causes.

Morbidity

- National and local registers provide data of variable accuracy. Registers exist for cancers (type of cancer, treatment, and survival), drug addiction, congenital abnormalities and specific diseases (such as diabetes and stroke) (www.nchod.org.uk).
- Communicable disease notification provides a source of information for local surveillance (www.hpa.org.uk).
- Information from the general medical services contract (quality and outcomes framework) provides morbidity data for certain disease groups (www.ic.nhs.uk).
- Prescribing data can be a valuable surrogate marker of morbidity.

Healthcare

- Hospital activity data can provide information on hospital admissions, diagnoses, length of stay, operations performed, and patients' characteristics) (www.nchod.org.uk; www.ic.nhs.uk).
- Clinical indicators such as the health service indicators, can provide information on the comparative performance of hospitals and health authorities (www.ic.nhs.uk).

Reproduced with permission from BMJ Publishing Group Ltd.[11]

> **Box 6.2** *Public involvement in health needs assessment[10]*
>
> *Some useful methods of public involvement*
>
> - Informal discussions
> - Interviews and focus groups with patients, users and carers
> - Surveys of patients, users and carers (paper, street, online)
> - Suggestion boxes
> - Feedback from complaints procedures
> - Contacts through online health forums and discussion groups
>
> *Sources of groups for consultation*
>
> - Local involvement networks (LINks)
> - Voluntary sector
> - Practice-based patient groups
> - Schools and colleges
> - Churches and community centres
> - Local employers

by the people affected by an issue or problem, by other people representing them, or by both groups together.

There are four key principles in advocacy.

- *Human rights:* health is recognised as a basic human right.
- *Democracy:* people within local communities should be and are encouraged and supported to participate in any decision making that impacts on health.
- *Inclusion:* partnership working ensures that people, communities and organisations are involved in planning and delivering services.
- *Equity:* resources must be distributed fairly, including opportunities to access and use services. Equitable distribution is based on need, not demand and is not the same as equal distribution. Equal distribution of resources could result in those with greatest need having insufficient, while those with the least need have excess. Inequitable distribution is unjust, unfair and may be unequal, but is also remediable. Much of public health practice focuses on ensuring equity to reduce inequalities.

Advocacy is often more powerful if those affected by the problem or issue are involved in or lead the process. This can sometimes be viewed as difficult to achieve and the differences in perspectives between patients and the public and healthcare providers hard to reconcile. However, advocacy or 'voice' is a crucial element in the context of undertaking HNAs and therefore, despite the difficulties, needs to be included.

Social marketing and social marketing insight

In recent years the concept of social marketing has been used in healthcare as a way of helping service commissioners to understand how and why people behave the way they do in terms of health behaviours (smoking, eating, taking physical activity, drinking, taking up screening or immunisation services) and why they access (or don't access) services to support a healthier lifestyle. Social marketing insight is essentially the technique involved in understanding attitudes and beliefs which lead people to behave in certain ways and what the barriers and facilitators are for supporting behaviour change. Social marketing (i.e. communicating a specific message in a way that it will be understood) can then be used to support behaviour change. The techniques used to determine attitudes and behaviours are also useful for obtaining people's views on how services can be established and managed. A programme called 'Health Insight'[15] seeks to use what is learnt about consumer behaviour to inform local and national health improvement activities through interventions which are better targeted to people at high risk of unhealthy lifestyles. Market research techniques are used to obtain this insight into behaviours and can also be used to determine what the public want from services aimed at improving health.[16,17]

Prioritisation of needs and services designed to meet needs

A needs assessment may identify a number of areas for development, but given limitations of resources, these may need to be prioritised. This can be very difficult. At a national level, organisations such as NICE use economic methods to indicate whether different initiatives should be supported (see Chapter 7). However, within local or focused HNA, prioritisation methods are much more subjective, although the process should ideally always involve service users and carers. Two contrasting methods are the use of ranking matrices and nominal groups. The former can be developed as a questionnaire, distributed to large sections of the population or to a wide number of stakeholders, whereas the latter is carried out during a face-to-face meeting, hence can involve only a small number of individuals.

Ranking matrices require the development of a scoring system that allocates different weights to different factors. The system can be highly complex but, if involving the public, needs to be relatively simple. The important factors must be identified and participants in the prioritisation process asked to rate each need or proposed service against each factor. Simple factors could be 'importance', 'feasibility' or 'likely cost'. Others are suggested in Table 6.2. A scale could be developed such as 1 (low) to 5 (high) for each factor and the scores summed to establish priorities. This process is usually conducted once, and inevitably there will be

Table 6.2 Factors useful for prioritising needs or services

Factor	Questions
Incidence/prevalence of the need	How common is it in the locality?
Capacity to benefit from a service	How many patients are likely to benefit?
Inequalities	How effectively will the service address inequalities?
NHS priorities/PCT workplan	Does the service address any national or local health priorities?
	Is the need identified within the JSNA?
Time to benefit	How long will it be before benefits are seen?
Effectiveness	Is there evidence to support a new service?
Cost-effectiveness/value for money	What is the cost of addressing the need?
	Is it worth it for the health gained?
Risk assessment	What are the risks of not meeting the need?
Public view	How important is the need in the public view?

Adapted from reference 18.
JSNA = joint strategic needs assessment

disagreements, therefore some method of deciding the level of agreement that is acceptable is required in advance.

To conduct a nominal group, all relevant stakeholders should be invited, which should include representatives of the public or patients and carers. The needs identified by the HNA are listed, discussed generally, then ranked individually by each participant. The discussion is in fact part of the process, since it can effectively change the views of individuals. The quantitative aspect derives from the ranking process. The results of the ranking are displayed to the group and the discussion re-started, followed by a second round of individual ranking. The process is continued until acceptable consensus is reached.

Health needs assessments within healthcare policy in England

The White Paper *Our Health, Our Care, Our Say*[19] set out clear directions for PCTs to work in partnership with local authority and other statutory bodies to improve the health and well-being of the local population. This policy also required directors of public health, adult social services and children's services to work collaboratively to identify local needs that could support the planning and commissioning of local services. The requirement was laid down in statute as a 'duty' to establish a joint strategic needs assessment (JSNA) and guidance provided on how this should be carried out and endorsed by the NHS Next Stage Review in 2008.[13] Different policies and processes are in place in the other home countries.

Joint strategic needs assessment

The JSNA describes 'a process of gathering intelligence (information) to help Local Authorities and PCTs commission services effectively and efficiently'.[20] In essence it identifies current and future health and well-being needs in the light of existing services and informs future service planning, taking into account evidence of effectiveness. In other words a JSNA describes 'the big picture' in terms of the health and well-being needs and inequalities for an entire local community for whom the NHS and local authority have a responsibility. This includes care groups, non-resident users and often non-registered groups, such as refugees and asylum seekers.

The JSNA should enable the understanding of health and well-being needs over the short term (three to five years) and over the longer term (five to ten years). These will then inform local area agreements and strategic planning within the locality. Agreements are negotiated between all the main public sector organisations (NHS, local government and police) within a geographical area (usually based on local government areas) and are designed to make the local organisations more accountable to local people. They are also aimed at helping to make services more 'joined up', to help organisations to work together to improve health (see Chapter 8). The JSNA supports the commissioning of services and interventions to improve health and well-being and reduce inequalities. The JSNA is also part of joint local working (see Chapter 8), which should enable the achievement of a wide range of outcomes considered important by government. The outcome-based approach is designed to allow local organisations to develop local solutions/services. The outcomes are listed in a national indicator set for local authorities and local partnerships and in the NHS performance indicators (Vital Signs). These indicators are linked not only to health and use of health services but also to the wider determinants of health.[21] The JSNA core data set uses these performance indicators to support PCTs to achieve the desired outcomes.

Key aims of the JSNA[20] are to:

- build on existing knowledge of the population and establish a picture of future needs
- develop a framework for active engagement of users and carers and the wider community, building on existing structures
- embed public health intelligence within the cycle of health service commissioning leading to more effective commissioning and decommissioning of services (Figure 6.2)

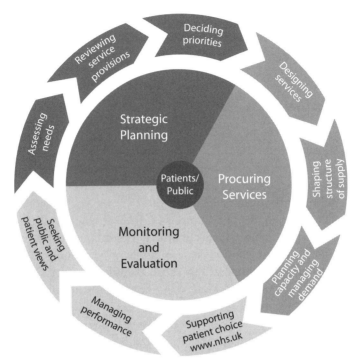

Figure 6.2 The World Class Commissioning cycle. Reproduced with permission from the NHS information centre.[22]

- shape the strategic direction of local area agreements and therefore the work of the wider partnership in tackling health inequalities (see Chapter 8)
- signal commissioning intentions to service providers (including voluntary sector providers) to support direction and development.

Using a joint strategic needs assessment to commission services

Once needs have been identified and prioritised, local teams within NHS organisations commission services to meet the needs. Historically there have been differences across the NHS, not only in the quality of services provided but also in the way they have been commissioned. The DoH established a programme called World Class Commissioning which included national standards for commissioning organisations to help them deliver/achieve better services and outcomes. Putting patients central to decision making ensures that there is a long term focus on prevention and health promotion. Two of the standards within World Class Commissioning were there to develop the JSNA to identify the local needs now and in the future and for PCTs to work with other partners[22,23] (see Chapter 8).

Health needs assessment within pharmacy

The principles of HNA require pharmacists to look at local mortality and morbidity profiles, examine the services they offer and consult with patients, carers and local healthcare professionals who also use their services, to help them identify services that need to be increased and improved as well as those that are not being used and can be stopped. Needs assessments can be undertaken by individual pharmacy organisations whether this is in primary care, community pharmacy or in hospitals. HNA ensures that pharmacists are providing the right services for the needs of the population they look after, and whether there are patients who are not receiving services that they need. However, it must be remembered that needs are not static and will change over time, therefore the process is clearly part of a cycle of improvement to identify needs and how these change. HNA should therefore be repeated at regular, albeit perhaps not frequent, intervals.

The method can be used to establish novel pharmaceutical services, for example, the Middlefield project (see Box 3.1) or adapted to prioritise services provided to a medical practice where the 'service users' are the staff working there.[24,25] Community pharmacists in particular should use HNA to identify ways in which they can develop and improve their services as well as contributing to the JSNA.

Pharmaceutical needs assessment

Most PCTs in England have undertaken a pharmaceutical needs assessment in recent years. The requirement to undertake an assessment has become more defined because of direction from the DoH, which will mean that, in future, the opening of new community pharmacies will become an integral part of the overall strategic planning and commissioning of services within PCTs. However, the breadth and depth of the assessments carried out and consistency of what was included has been variable.[26] New guidance has therefore been published[18] which provides a consistent structure for the pharmaceutical needs assessment, requiring it to be integrated with the JSNA.

Local community pharmacists must be involved in the process and help to influence service development, although assessments are likely to be led by PCTs. Data gathering is clearly important and includes obtaining the views of patients and the public. As part of their contract with the NHS, all community pharmacists are required to conduct annual surveys of their NHS customers to assess satisfaction with services. Although there are standard templates available for this,[27] more specific, detailed questions can be added, to provide valuable information for the purposes of assessment, but additional methods of involving the public should also be used. Most surveys are aimed at existing users of services but, to obtain the views of potential service users, standard market research methods such as street surveys, telephone surveys and postal questionnaires could be used.[28,29]

As part of a pharmaceutical needs assessment, PCTs have to prioritise needs, map need against existing service provision (see Table 6.3) and then establish the willingness of pharmacists to provide specific services. PCTs will then seek to commission services from pharmacists. Specialist public health pharmacists are likely to be involved in these processes, whereas community pharmacists need to be involved in developing and delivering the services. Chapter 9 describes service development in more detail.

Table 6.3 Mapping service need to service provision

Mapping by identified public health need

Identified need	Pharmacy services	Other relevant services	Gap between need and provision
Rates of CHD are higher in areas of highest deprivation within the PCT	Most offer smoking cessation advice, but none offer CHD screening	One GP practice currently offering routine CHD screening	Limited provision of CHD screening

Mapping by target

Target/priority	Pharmacy services	Other relevant services	Gaps
Reduce hospital admissions related to alcohol	None currently provided	Staff from some medical practices have received training in brief interventions and refer patients to relevant secondary services	Pharmacists could provide brief interventions and referral

Mapping by locality

Locality	Identified need	Pharmacy services meeting need	Improvements required
Highly deprived area within the PCT	Residents have limited access to both GP and pharmacy services	Nearest pharmacy (2.4 km) requires crossing dual carriageway by bridge	New pharmacy service providing NHS dispensing, public health advice and OTC medicines

Mapping by service

Service	Need	Current service available	Gaps
Free provision of EHC to under 18 year olds	Some areas have limited access to any service	Selected pharmacies and family planning clinics (latter not open at weekends)	Increased availability of service through pharmacies

Adapted from reference 18.
CHD = coronary heart disease; PCT = primary care trust; GP = general practitioner; OTC = over-the-counter;
EHC = emergency hormonal contraception.

References

1. Stevens A, Raferty J, Mant J *et al. Health Care Needs Assessment: The epidemiologically based needs assessment reviews,* 2nd ed. Oxford: Radcliffe Medical Press, 2004.
2. Wright J, Williams R, Wilkinson JR. Development of the importance of the Health Needs Assessment. *BMJ* 1998; 316: 1310–1313 (25 April).
3. Department of Health. *The Health of the Nation: A strategy for health in England.* London: HMSO, 1992.
4. Shanks J, Kheraj S, Fish S. Better ways of assessing health needs in primary care. *BMJ* 1995; 310: 480–481.
5. Tudor Hart J. The inverse care law. *Lancet* 1971; i: 405–412.
6. Culyer AJ. *Need and the National Health Service.* London: Martin Robertson, 1976.
7. Williams R. Priorities not needs. In: Corden A, Robertson G, Tolley K, eds. *Meeting needs.* Aldershot: Avebury Gower, 1992.
8. Stevens A, Gabbay J. Needs Assessment, needs assessment. *Health Trends* 1991; 23: 20–23.
9. Donaldson C, Mooney G. Needs assessment, priority setting, and contracts for health care: an economic view. *BMJ* 1991; 303: 1529–1530.
10. Wilkinson JR, Murray SA. Health Needs Assessment. Assessment in primary care: practical issues and possible approaches. *BMJ* 1998; 316: 1524–1528 (16 May).
11. Based on information in Williams R, Wright J. Health Needs Assessment: epidemiological issues in health needs assessment. *BMJ* 1998; 316: 1379–1382.
12. Examples of the policy documents on patient and public involvement can be found at http://www.dh.gov.uk/en/Managingyourorganisation/PatientAndPublicinvolvement/DH_08587.
13. Department of Health. *High Quality Care For All: NHS next stage review – final report.* London: DoH, July 2008. http://www.dh.gov.uk/en/Publicationsandstatistics/Publications/PublicationsPolicyAndGuidance/DH_085825.
14. National Centre for Involvement. *Local Involvement Networks.* http://www.nhscentreforinvolvement.nhs.uk/index.cfm?content=110.
15. Department of Health. *Ambitions for Health: A strategic framework for maximising the potential of social marketing and health-related behaviour.* London: Department of Health, 2008. http://www.dh.gov.uk/en/Publichealth/Choosinghealth/DH_066342.
16. Department of Health. *Self-care: A national view in 2007 compared to 2003–2004.* London: Department of Health, 2008.
17. Patients Association. *2008 Community pharmacist – here to help.*
18. NHS Employers. *Developing Pharmaceutical Needs Assessments: A practical guide.* 2009. http://www.nhsemployers.org/SiteCollectionDocuments/Combined%20final%20PNA_140709_af.pdf.
19. Department of Health. *Our Health, Our Care, Our Say.* London: Department of Health, 2006.
20. Department of Health. *Guidance on Joint Strategic Needs Assessment.* London: Department of Health, 2007.
21. HM Government. *The New Performance Framework for Local Authorities and Local Authority Partnerships: Single set of national indicators.* http://www.communities.gov.uk/publications/localgovernment/nationalindicator.
22. The Information Centre. *World-Class Commissioning Cycle.* http://www.ic.nhs.uk/commissioning.
23. Department of Health. *World Class Commissioning Vision.* 2007. http://www.dh.gov.uk/en/Publicationsandstatistics/Publications/PublicationsPolicyAndguidance/DH_080956. London: Department of Health, 2007.
24. Krska J, Duffus PRS. Pharmaceutical needs assessment in general practice. *Int J Pharm Pract* 2000; 8: 265–274.
25. Krska J, Ross SM. Prioritising the work of a practice pharmacist. *Pharmacy Pract* 2002; 12: 101–106.

26. Elvey R, Bradley F, Ashcroft D *et al.* Commissioning services and the new pharmacy contract (1) pharmaceutical needs assessment and the uptake of new pharmacy contract. *Pharm J* 2006; 277: 161–163.

27. Pharmaceutical Services Negotiating Committee. *Community Pharmacy Patient Questionnaire.* 2009. http://www.psnc.org.uk/pages/community_pharmacy_patient_questionnaire_cppq.html

28. Krska J *et al.* Weight management services in community pharmacy: identifying opportunities. *Int J Pharm Pract* 2010; 18: 7–12.

29. Krska J, Morecroft CW. Views of the general public on the role of pharmacy in public health. *J Pharm Health Serv Res* 2010; 1: 33–38.

Suggested reading

National Institute for Health and Clinical Excellence. *Health Needs Assessment: A practical Guide.* London: NICE, 2010. http://www.nice.org.uk/media/150/35/Health_Needs_Assessment_A_Practical_Guide.pdf.

7

Evidence-based delivery

Dyfrig A Hughes

Evidence-based medicine

The origins of evidence-based medicine (EBM) date to the early 1990s, when Guyatt, Sackett and others at McMaster University, Ontario, Canada developed practical methodologies to implement concepts described earlier by Archie Cochrane in his book *Effectiveness and Efficiency: Random reflections on health services*, published in 1972.[1] The basic principle of EBM – that we should treat where there is evidence of benefit and not treat where there is evidence of no benefit (or harm) – makes explicit the importance of evidence in arriving at the most appropriate choice of treatment. EBM has been formally defined as 'the conscientious, explicit, and judicious use of current best evidence in making decisions about the care of individual patients.'[2] Note the emphasis here is on individuals, not populations; however, EBM does apply to both (see page 113 and Chapter 14).

The importance of basing treatment decisions on robust scientific evidence, and not on conventional wisdom, can be exemplified with the routine practice of administering intravenous corticosteroids for patients who experienced cerebral oedema as a consequence of head injury. In the 1990s the UK Medical Research Council funded the CRASH trial to test whether this practice was indeed beneficial. The trial recruited about 10 000 patients – it was designed to recruit 20 000 worldwide but was terminated early as it showed an increase in the risk of death (3% higher in absolute terms and 18% higher in relative terms) in the group of patients receiving steroids. Steroid infusion was expected to reduce death and disability but the trial evidence showed convincingly that it did not.[3] The ill-founded use of corticosteroids, without supporting evidence of effectiveness, has been estimated to have contributed to the deaths of 75 000 people worldwide.

A second example is that of a missed opportunity for earlier routine use of an effective therapy because of a lack of a systematic review and analysis of existing data. Intravenous streptokinase became standard therapy for acute myocardial infarction following its approval by regulatory authorities in the 1990s. However, it transpired that, had a systematic review and meta-analysis been performed, there was sufficient evidence to support its use as a life-saving intervention 20 years earlier.[4]

There are a number of stark examples such as these, and countless others, where patient care might not have been optimised owing to a lack of an evidence-based approach. These examples also illustrate the different forms of evidence that can be used to inform a decision or policy on the use of medicines. Indeed, there is a range of epidemiological methods that can be used to assess the effect of treatments (see Chapter 4 and Table 7.1). There are advantages and disadvantages to each. Whereas the randomised controlled trial (RCT) is seen as the 'gold standard' approach for the

Table 7.1 Common study methods used to assess the effects of treatment

Study type	Feature
Case report	These are reports on single patients. Because they are reports of cases and use no control groups with which to compare outcomes, they have no statistical validity
Case series	These consist of collections of reports on the treatment of individual patients
Case control studies	These are studies in which patients who already have a specific condition are compared with people who do not. These types of studies are often less reliable than RCT, and cohort studies for the assessment of efficacy/effectiveness because showing a statistical relationship does not mean that one factor necessarily caused the other
Cohort studies	These take a large population and follow patients who have a specific condition or receive a particular treatment over time and compare them with another group that is similar but has not been affected by the condition being studied. Cohort studies are not as reliable as RCTs for the assessment of efficacy/effectiveness, since the two groups may differ in ways other than in the variable under study
Randomised controlled trials	These include methodologies that reduce the potential for bias and allow for comparison between intervention groups and control groups. This is considered to be the 'gold standard' approach to assessing the efficacy of effectiveness of treatment
Systematic reviews	These usually focus on a clinical topic and answer a specific question. Extensive literature searches are conducted to identify studies with sound methodology. The studies are reviewed, assessed, and summarised according to the predetermined criteria of the review question
Meta-analyses	These take the systematic review a step further by using statistical techniques to combine the results of several studies as if they were one large study

assessment of efficacy and effectiveness, a cohort study might be more practical and appropriate for rare adverse drug reactions.

The level of confidence that can be placed on the inferences made from such studies can be ranked from high to low, as follows:

- high quality meta-analyses, systematic reviews of RCTs, or RCTs with a very low risk of bias
- well-conducted meta-analyses, systematic reviews, or RCTs with a low risk of bias
- meta-analyses, systematic reviews, or RCTs with a high risk of bias
- high quality systematic reviews of case control or cohort or studies
- high quality case control or cohort studies with a very low risk of confounding or bias and a high probability that the relationship is causal
- well-conducted case control or cohort studies with a low risk of confounding or bias and a moderate probability that the relationship is causal
- case control or cohort studies with a high risk of confounding or bias and a significant risk that the relationship is not causal
- non-analytic studies, e.g. case reports, case series
- expert opinion.

A difficulty for healthcare professionals is to distil the evidence into manageable pieces to inform practice. Several thousand research studies are published each year, making it impossible for pharmacists to keep abreast of the evidence. To address the need for evidence-based practice, organisations such as the Cochrane Collaboration (www.cochrane.org), NICE (www.nice.org.uk) and the Scottish Intercollegiate Guidelines Network (SIGN, www.sign.ac.uk) produce and disseminate reviews and clinical guidelines of best practice. Syntheses of evidence can be accessed via the NHS Evidence search portal at www.evidence.nhs.uk, the Cochrane Library at www.thecochranelibrary.com and the Cochrane Database of Systematic Reviews, the TRIP (Turning Research Into Practice) Database (www.tripdatabase.com) and the Database of Abstracts of Reviews of Effectiveness (DARE, www.crd.york.ac.uk). Additionally, there are dedicated journals, including *Health Technology Assessment* and *Evidence-based Medicine*, as well as general medical and clinical speciality journals, that publish primary as well as secondary (review) evidence.

These are normally the first ports of call for pharmacists seeking evidence on aspects of a treatment in question. However, despite their increasing coverage and comprehensiveness, there will be occasions when a formal EBM approach is necessary. To be confident in the conclusions of any review or guideline, practising pharmacists need to be satisfied that rigorous EBM methods have been followed. The skills of critical appraisal are essential to enable effective implementation of scientific findings to practice.

The methods of EBM encompass the specification of a question for which an evidence-based answer is sought, the identification of the relevant information sources and the synthesis and interpretation of the data. EBM is about making best use of existing data to inform decisions, and the processes followed can be summarised by the following steps[5]:

1   converting the need of information into an answerable question
2   tracking down the best evidence with which to answer that question
3   critically appraising that evidence for its validity, impact and applicability
4   integrating the critical appraisal with clinical expertise and with patient's unique biology, values and circumstances
5   evaluating the effectiveness and efficiency in executing steps 1 to 4 and seeking ways to improve them both in the future.

Formulating an evidence-based medicine question

When faced with decisions, such as the prescribing of a medicine in individual patients, the selection of medicines for inclusion in a formulary, or appraisal by a regional or national health technology appraisal body, the starting point is to formulate a question that can be answered from the available evidence. The *PICOt* model (*P*opulation, *I*ntervention, *C*omparison, *O*utcome, *t*ime) is a useful system for this purpose (Table 7.2).

Table 7.2 Summary of the PICOt model for specifying the evidence-based medicine question

Factor	Ask yourself:
Population (patient/condition)	What is the principal indication for therapy? What are the most important characteristics of the patient? This may include the primary problem, disease, or co-existing conditions. Consider important demographic variables such as gender and age. Are there particular subgroups that need to be considered?
Intervention (drug/dose, procedure, diagnostic test)	Which drug (or combination of drugs) and which dose, regimen and dosage form?
Comparison	What is the main alternative to compare with the intervention? It might be an active comparator (e.g. representative of routine care) no medication or placebo
Outcome	What can be accomplished, measured, improved or affected? What is the goal of therapy for the patient? Relieve or eliminate the symptoms? Reduce the number of adverse events? Improve function or test scores? Improve health-related quality of life? Or life expectancy?
Time	Each variable needs a temporal element. How old are the participants? How long is the treatment given for? When is the outcome measured?

Choosing the right outcomes

It is important to consider the relevance of evidence according to the outcome being measured – whether the focus is on patient oriented outcomes, or some disease-oriented outcome. Evidence derived from the former are often referred to as POEMs (patient-oriented evidence that matters) and the latter as DOEs (disease-oriented evidence). A study addressing health related quality-of-life issues, mortality and morbidity is called a POEM. Studies classified as POEMs use patient-related outcome measures and may lead healthcare professionals to alter their patterns of practice. A study addressing factors such as organ function, biochemical changes, or pharmacodynamics is called a DOE study. Our knowledge and understanding of aetiology, prevalence, pathophysiology and pharmacology is enhanced by the DOE study, but they have less direct relevance to patients. Consider a new treatment for osteoporosis. A DOE might be the increase in bone mineral density, whereas an outcome measure is the reduced risk to patients of fracture. Although bone mineral density is predictive of fracture risk, it is no substitute for direct measurement of fracture rates. A drug that improves bone density might not necessarily reduce the risk of fractures in osteoporotic patients. The same is true of cholesterol-lowering agents: low density lipoprotein (LDL) cholesterol is a predictor of cardiac events, but a study that only measures serum LDL cannot be regarded as being sufficient to conclude that a particular drug increases life-expectancy. To the practitioner of EBM, studies that provide POEMs are of more relevance than those focusing on DOEs.

This can be illustrated with examples where, against expectations, DOEs do not translate to outcome measures. One such case was in relation to the antiarrhythmic drugs flecainide and encainide. Both are highly effective in suppressing the ventricular premature contractions that occur following a myocardial infarction, and were used extensively (200 000 persons per year in the United States) in the belief that this would translate to better outcomes for patients. A trial called the Cardiac Arrhythmia Suppression Trial was set up to test whether either drug (and a third, moricizine) improved survival in over 2300 patients.[6] The result was startling. Rather than saving lives, flecainide and encainide actually increased the risk of death by causing the cardiac arrests the drugs were supposed to prevent. There were 63 sudden deaths in the encainide and flecainide group, compared with 26 in the placebo group. Later, an increased risk for death in patients receiving moricizine was also established. The trial was stopped prematurely and the use of these drugs curtailed.

Returning to osteoporosis, sodium fluoride stimulates bone formation and increases bone mass. It came into widespread use, although it was not approved by the regulatory authorities. A four-year, placebo-controlled, randomised trial of fluoride in 202 postmenopausal women who had osteoporosis and vertebral fractures confirmed that treatment increased bone mineral density in the lumbar spine by 35%.[7] However, the trial also showed that new vertebral fractures occurred significantly more frequently in patients treated with fluoride than in those who received placebo (163 compared with 136 fractures). The same was observed for non-vertebral fractures.

For all the right reasons, therefore, evidence-based practice should be underpinned by evidence, reporting outcomes that are of importance to patients, and not to experimental scientists.

Accessing and analysing the evidence

As mentioned earlier, a PICOt question might be answered adequately by an existing resource such as a NICE guideline. However, to best illustrate how to answer a PICOt question from first principles, it is important to be familiar with the steps that are followed by systematic reviewers – the professional evidence synthesisers.

The first step is to translate a clearly and precisely specified PICOt question into appropriate search terms for interrogating databases of medical literature. Electronic databases, such as Medline (PubMed, www.ncbi.nlm.nih.gov/pubmed), Embase and the Cochrane Library, catalogue published articles that are most likely to be relevant for retrieval of evidence related to the PICOt question. To be systematic, a literature search should cover a range of sources, as they tend to include different journals or types of articles. A rigorous review will identify relevant articles from the 'grey' literature – unpublished articles and conference proceedings, and by hand-searching key journals as well as asking opinion leaders for evidence they may be aware of. This is important as only half of RCTs presented at conferences are ever published. It is usual for searches to be limited to articles published in the English language, but this might lead to bias if relevant articles in other languages are missed – about half of all trials in physiotherapy are not in English. The period that the search should cover will depend on the nature of the medicine under consideration. For a new medicine, it is clearly unlikely that much published evidence will be available at the launch date. For others, it may be appropriate to limit the search to five or ten years, or longer, as necessary.

Organisations, such as the Cochrane Collaboration, have developed standard search strategies to identify relevant articles, according to type, such as meta-analyses, systematic reviews, RCTs and so on. Although useful, these and other search filters are not perfect. Some studies will be missed and many irrelevant studies will be identified. The search strategy can be tailored to adjust the balance between sensitivity and specificity, so as to avoid an unmanageable number of 'hits' while keeping the number of missed articles to a minimum.

Before any papers are acquired for evaluation, the next step is sifting of the search outputs, to eliminate duplicate citations and material that is clearly irrelevant. This is normally done on the basis of the title and content of the abstract and is performed according to a pre-defined set of inclusion and exclusion criteria by two or more researchers independently to avoid any selection bias. Any disagreements are normally resolved through discussion. Only then are the full text articles retrieved and a second review conducted in the same manner. From the final listing of studies, relevant data on the population, methods, intervention, outcome measures, results, statistical significance, authors' conclusions and so on, are then extracted on to a standardised form.

Extracted data may be synthesised qualitatively or quantitatively. A qualitative (narrative) overview of the clinical evidence is helpful but less useful than a quantitative approach. The latter, where feasible, improves the statistical power of detecting any difference between treatment and control. Individual studies might not in themselves be sufficiently large to detect small differences in outcome, but a meta-analysis of many such trials enables the pooling of results from several comparable RCTs to increase the power to detect small differences. When each individual trial included in a meta-analysis is of high quality and there is no evidence of publication bias, it is not surprising that meta-analyses are among the preferred evidence source for EBM.

Meta-analyses are not always appropriate, however. Trials may vary in terms of types of patient, treatment, methodology and outcomes etc. This may cause variability from trial to trial in the estimate of the effect of the medicine. This is called heterogeneity (which may be statistical or clinical) and may make pooling of data in meta-analysis unreliable or inappropriate.

Critical appraisal

Critical appraisal is the process of carefully and systematically examining research to judge its validity and its value and relevance in a particular context. It is an essential skill for EBM because it allows practising pharmacists to assess whether a study is relevant and, importantly, whether the study's results could be biased. A useful and systematic approach to critical appraisal is to follow a checklist. Standard checklists cover a number of research methods, and one that is applicable for RCTs is reproduced in Box 7.1. Trials not adhering to the methods of standard reporting (CONSORT: Consolidated Standards of Reporting Trials[8]) should be viewed with suspicion.

Box 7.1 *Checklist for the quality assessment of randomised controlled trials in evidence-based medicine**

Step 1: Are the results valid?

1 Was the assignment of patients to treatments randomised?
2 Was randomisation list concealed? Can you tell?
3 Were all the subjects who entered the trial accounted for at its conclusion?
4 Were they analysed in the groups to which they were randomised, i.e. intention-to-treat analysis?
5 Were patients, researchers and clinicians 'blind' to which treatment was being received, i.e. could they tell?
6 Aside from the experimental treatment, were the groups treated equally?
7 Were the groups similar at the start of the trial (e.g. with respect to demographic and prognostic factors)?

Step 2: What are the results?

1 How large was the treatment effect?
   • How were the results expressed? (RRR, NNT, etc.)
2 How precise were the results?
   • Were the results presented with confidence intervals?

Step 3: How can I apply these results to my patient?

1 Do these results apply to my patient?
   • Consider PICOt – *p*atients, *i*ntervention, *c*omparison, *o*utcome(s) and *t*ime
   • Is my patient so different from those in the trial that the results don't apply?
   • How great would the benefit of therapy be for my particular patient?
2 Are my patient's values and preferences satisfied by the intervention offered?
   • Do I have a clear assessment of my patient's values and preferences?
   • Are they met by this regimen and its potential consequences?

*Adapted from *Critical Appraisal Skills Programme (CASP)*, Public Health Resource Unit, Institute of Health Science, Oxford; Guyatt GH, Sackett DL, Cook DJ. Users guides to the medical literature. II. How to use an article about therapy or prevention. A. Are the results of the study valid? *JAMA* 1993; 270: 2598–2601; Guyatt GH, Sackett DL, Cook DJ. Users guides to the medical literature. II. How to use an article about therapy or prevention. B. What were the results and will they help me in caring for my patients? *JAMA* 1993; 271: 59–63.

There are three steps to critically appraise a RCT:

Step 1: Validity – are the study results valid? Were the methods appropriate?

Securing unbiased methods is essential for both correct attribution of cause to effect and estimate of the size of treatment effect.[9] Arguably the most important methodological component of trials is that of randomisation. It is the process of assigning patients to study groups based on chance. Without the random element, for instance, if trialists allocated patients according to their age (odd/even), dates of birth or other similar method, there is potential for selection bias being introduced. Randomisation is based on computer-generated random numbers and ensures that both known and unknown factors (known as risk or prognostic factors) are balanced. Non-randomised controlled trials can detect associations between an intervention and an outcome, but they cannot rule out the possibility that the association was caused by a third factor linked to both intervention and outcome. According to the CONSORT statement, trials are required to report randomisation methods, and the absence of information on randomisation does not guarantee that adequate and reliable methods have been employed. Concealed randomisation means preventing the prescribing clinician and others involved in the trial from identifying the treatment groups to which patients are assigned. If they were able to do so, they may be inclined to allocate the treatment they considered to be most effective to sicker patients, thereby introducing bias. Randomisation may be concealed by use of opaque envelopes or, more often nowadays, central telephone or web-based patient randomisation systems and services.

The results section of clinical trials should report the baseline characteristics of patients, according to the treatment group to which they were allocated. Any imbalance between groups is a warning of improper randomisation for, if a prognostic factor (e.g. age, disease severity, renal function) differs, there is good likelihood for bias.

Double blinding ensures that the preconceived views of patients and clinicians cannot systematically bias the assessment of outcomes. However, it is not fool proof – treatment identification may be exposed to researchers and/or patients because of the unique action of a drug such as dry mouth, or more obvious still, coloured urine as in the case of rifampicin and some other drugs. In a systematic review of 250 studies, it was noted that, compared with trials in which authors reported adequately concealed treatment allocation, trials in which concealment was either inadequate or unclear yielded significantly larger estimates of treatment effects. Odds ratios were exaggerated by as much as 41%.[10] Sometimes blinding is not possible for practical reasons (e.g. a trial comparing four alternative medicines will require multiple placebo dummies to maintain blinding, but patients might consequently be non-adherent). An unblinded trial is described as an 'open label' trial.

Intention-to-treat analysis refers to the analysis of the trial according to the treatment groups to which patients were allocated, not to what they might ultimately receive. Within trials, patients may be permitted to switch treatments, or they might fail to complete or take their medication. In such cases, an analysis based on what they ultimately received (known as per protocol analysis) could be biased. For instance, if patients failed to respond to the treatment to which they were initially assigned, a per protocol analysis will produce a falsely high estimate of treatment effect.

The attribution of effect to the treatment in question requires that all other factors are kept constant, or in other words, the only difference between the experimental arms of the trial is the treatment. Any additional change might introduce bias. This can be controlled through blinding.

For one reason or another, some patients invariably withdraw, or 'drop out' of trials. This may be due to adverse effects, lack of response (or responding well), non-adherence, change in personal circumstances, etc. There is an important difference, however, between dropping out of assigned treatment and dropping out of the trial altogether (e.g. patient withdraws consent). It is essential that trialists follow up patients the best they can, to gain an understanding (for instance) of whether a particular treatment was not very effective. 'Lost to follow-up' is uninformative and compromises the validity of the study.

Step 2: What are the results?

The interpretation of the results of a clinical trial requires knowledge of measures of treatment effect, such as odds ratios, hazard ratios and numbers needed to treat; and basic statistics. A glossary of the most commonly used measures is provided in Table 7.3.

During trial design, medical statisticians calculate the number of patients required to demonstrate some statistically and clinically significant difference between the treatment of interest, and the comparator. Power refers to the probability that a clinical trial will have a statistically significant result (usually p-value of less than 0.05). This probability is computed under the assumption that the treatment difference equals the minimally important difference – usually based on what is clinically meaningful.

The precision of the estimate of treatment effect is captured by the confidence interval – the range within which the true treatment effect is likely to lie (usually 95%) of the time. This provides information on whether or not the result of the trial is statistically significant. A trial that reports a relative risk reduction in stroke of 2% (and a 95% confidence interval spanning −0.5% to 4%) suggests that, although the study detected a reduction in relative risk of 2%, the true reduction could lie anywhere between −0.5% (i.e. an increase in risk) and 4%. When the 95% confidence interval spans zero, the trial does not provide convincing evidence that the treatment is effective.

Table 7.3 Commonly used measures of treatment effect

Measure	Definition
Odds ratio (OR)	A measure of treatment effectiveness. It is the odds of an event happening in the experimental group expressed as a proportion of the odds of an event happening in the control group. The closer the OR is to one, the smaller the difference in effect between the experimental intervention and the control intervention. If the OR is greater (or less) than one, then the effects of the treatment are more (or less) than those of the control treatment. It is calculated as the ratio of events to non-events in the intervention group over the ratio of events to non-events in the control group
Relative risk (RR)	The number of times more likely (RR >1) or less likely (RR <1) an event is to happen in one group compared with another. It is the ratio of the absolute risk (AR) for each group. It is analogous to the odds ratio (OR) when events are rare. Relative risk is defined as the absolute risk (AR) in the intervention group divided by the AR in the control group
Relative risk reduction (RRR)	The proportional reduction in risk between experimental and control participants in a trial. It is the complement of the relative risk (1 − RR)
Absolute risk (AR)	The probability that an individual will experience the specified outcome during a specified period. It lies in the range 0 to 1, or is expressed as a percentage
Absolute risk reduction (ARR)	The absolute difference in risk between the experimental and control groups in a trial. It is used when the risk in the control group exceeds the risk in the experimental group and is calculated by subtracting the AR in the experimental group (AR_{exp}) from the AR in the control group (AR_{cont})
Number needed to treat (NNT)	A measure of treatment effectiveness. It is the average number of people who need to be treated with a specific intervention for a given period of time to prevent one additional adverse outcome or achieve one additional beneficial outcome. NNT is calculated as 1/ARR. For a given outcome over a defined period of time, the lower the NNT, the more effective the treatment
Number needed to harm (NNH)	A measure of treatment harm. It is the average number of people from a defined population you would need to treat with a specific intervention for a given period of time to cause one additional adverse outcome. NNH can be calculated as $1/(AR_{exp} − AR_{cont})$
Hazard ratio (HR)	A measure of treatment effectiveness. Broadly equivalent to relative risk (RR); useful when the risk is not constant with respect to time. It uses information collected at different times. It is typically used in the context of survival over time. If the HR is 0.5 then the relative risk of dying in one group is half the risk of dying in the other group

Adapted from *Clinical Evidence* glossary. Reproduced with permission from the BMJ Publishing Group. (Source Clinical Evidence Online. www.clinicalevidence.bmj.com/ceweb/resources/glossary.jsp).

Step 3: How can I apply these results to my patient?

In essence, the more similar the study patients are to your patient, then the more applicable the study results are going to be. This relates to the PICOt criteria described earlier: if the demographic and clinical characteristics are comparable and the intervention is the same (drug, dose and regimen), then there is good likelihood that the results of the clinical trial may be generalisable – in other words there is sufficient external validity. If, on the other hand, trial patients are younger and have no or minimal co-morbidities, then the external validity is poor in relation to a patient who might be elderly with other medical conditions requiring concomitant therapy, and the trial results might not apply.

Randomised controlled trials tend to confirm a treatment's efficacy (whether it works), whereas the clinical question that matters relates to effectiveness (whether a treatment works in practice). Efficacy trials of pharmaceuticals usually compare a treatment with placebo, in a trial population that is carefully selected (usually male, otherwise healthy, not too old nor too young) and closely monitored, (e.g. require demonstration of adequate adherence prior to admission to the trial). These are the optimal conditions to show the maximum effect that a treatment might achieve (high internal validity), but these conditions differ substantially from what might be encountered in routine practice. Pragmatic trials are more appropriate for addressing issues of effectiveness as they tend to be more inclusive, compare treatments against usual practice, and therefore have greater external validity.

If the results of the evidence are relevant, unbiased, and trustworthy, the next step, and the most important step of the EBM framework, is to implement them in practice.

Implementing the evidence

Incorporating critical appraisal and EBM in practice is challenging. There are many barriers, such as time considerations and the fact that most research does not provide a clear-cut result. There is also risk of complacency – leaving it to NICE and others to pass judgement, but as NICE guidance only cover a small proportion of healthcare interventions, there will always be questions needing an answer through EBM. Furthermore, evidence-based practice changes over time. As new evidence becomes available, the relative place of treatments in therapy will change.

Critical appraisal skills improve with practice. Not only will this allow pharmacists to quickly separate the wheat from the chaff, but it will also encourage focusing their attention on the important sections of published studies and forming their own opinions instead of relying on those of the authors.

Despite the common sense approach of EBM, there remains a significant implementation problem, which is still variable in practice. For example, a study of guidelines issued by NICE found the impact on prescribing practice and use of evidence-based interventions was variable.[11] A more recent report[12] which detailed a study that compared the use of a selection of medicines as predicted by NICE, with actual use also showed high variance. Out of the 12 appraisals where a comparison could be made, observed use by the NHS in England was higher than predicted for seven, and lower for five. Both over- and under-use might be indicative of poor implementation, but could be attributed to other factors too. Research from the US suggests that only about 50% of interventions that should have been used by physicians according to evidence-based guidelines were actually prescribed.[13]

Dealing with competing priorities to ensure equitable distribution of services and technologies

Medicines whose harm/benefit profiles are favourable and for which there is evidence of effectiveness that is superior to existing therapy, might be seen as logical candidates for widespread use by the NHS. However, as is the case with many other health systems internationally, consideration of the treatment's cost-effectiveness (value for money) is necessary to ensure efficient use of the finite resources available for healthcare.

The NHS organisations within the four countries of the UK are committed to the principle that 'if you are ill or injured, there will be a national health service there to help and it will be based on need and need alone'. However, NHS trusts have a statutory requirement (under the 1977 NHS Act) to ensure that their expenditure does not exceed their income. Clearly these two commitments could conflict; careful judgement is required to balance them. Finite healthcare budgets dictate that we pay attention to costs as well as to needs. Hence, cost-effectiveness becomes important, as the best treatment for an individual might not necessarily be the best for populations or society. Suppose that £1 million is available for a vaccination programme and two potential vaccines are available: vaccine A is 95% effective, and costs £5 per dose, while vaccine B is 99% effective but is twice the cost. Individuals might reasonably prefer B. However, from a payer's perspective, £1 million would buy 200 000 doses of vaccine A and offer protection to 190 000 patients. Given the budget available, only 100 000 doses of the more effective vaccine B can be purchased, to protect 99 000 individuals. Thus, when costs are considered, the more effective intervention (for the individual) is inferior (from a population perspective) as only about half the number of people are given protection. The same principle applies to all health technologies, procedures, services and interventions.

Decisions on the availability and use of new medicines are made at various levels in the NHS, from national, through regional to local (see Chapter 14). There is therefore the potential for duplication of effort, significant differences in the conclusions reached and hence inequalities in the provision of care across the country (so-called 'postcode prescribing'). Evaluating technologies at a national level has the potential to reduce inequality and generally results in a very high standard of assessment; however, currently not all drugs and technologies are covered, deliberations can take a long time to become available and local affordability remains problematic.

Decisions about new medicines are based initially on considerations of clinical effectiveness and then on cost-effectiveness. The purpose of assessing cost-effectiveness is to inform decision-makers of the balance between costs and health gains, in order that health outcomes are maximised in the population. The aim is to minimise the [lost] opportunity cost, which is the value of the next best alternative that is foregone as the result of the decision.

Estimates of cost-effectiveness are derived from economic evaluations, which are comparative analyses of two or more therapeutic strategies in terms of their costs and consequences. 'Cost' is the sum of the number of individual resource items that are used, each multiplied by its unit costs. 'Consequences' are the health outcomes, for example, the impact of therapy on mortality or quality of life (or both).

Economic evaluation

All techniques of economic evaluation involve the same explicit consideration and calculation of the use of resources and overall costs. However, each method of evaluation handles consequences differently.

In health economics, the notion of cost is based on the value that would be gained from using resources elsewhere – referred to as the opportunity cost. In other words, resources used for one medicine are subsequently not available for use for other treatments or interventions and, as a result, the benefits that would have been derived have been sacrificed. Within economic evaluations, it is normally assumed that the price paid is a fair reflection of the opportunity cost. The principal categories of costs are:

- *direct costs,* which can be further categorised to medical costs (e.g. costs of treatment, cost of staff time, diagnostic tests, equipment) and patient costs (e.g. out-of-pocket costs for over-the-counter medicines, transport to and from hospital)
- *indirect costs,* including the costs of lost productivity through absence from work
- *intangible costs,* which are the most difficult to attach monetary value. They include the pain and suffering that may be associated with treatment (e.g. adverse drug reactions).

The perspective of an economic evaluation determines which costs are to be valued. The perspective might be narrow (e.g. a hospital) or broad (e.g. the NHS or society). It is not just the cost of the intervention that is subject to economic evaluation, but the total costs related to treatment with that intervention, including for instance hospitalisation, other interventions, blood tests and visits to GPs.

Medicines and other health care interventions often incur costs over a number of years, and so timing is an important factor in many costings and is accounted for in several ways. First, all costs are valued in a base year, which normally reflects the latest available prices. Secondly, capital costs are apportioned over the lifetime of the item (e.g. building, substantial equipment). Thirdly, future costs are discounted back to the base year. In general terms, this reflects a preference by people to put off costs rather than to pay immediately. NICE currently discounts both costs and benefits at 3.5% per annum.

Cost-minimisation analysis

Cost-minimisation analysis (CMA) requires robust evidence to show that two or more interventions have exactly the same health effects, i.e. are therapeutically equivalent in terms of health benefits and adverse effects. It could be used to compare branded and generic medicines, or different formulations of the same drug, but its practical applications are limited. However, in the absence of access to economic and health outcome data, many decisions made at local level are based (inappropriately) on CMA, primarily the acquisition or purchasing costs of drugs.

Cost-effectiveness analysis

Cost-effectiveness analysis (CEA) is appropriate when the sizes of the health effects of two or more interventions are not identical, but are measured in the same units, e.g. life-years gained or reduction in LDL cholesterol. They are used to address issues of technical efficiency. Technical efficiency answers questions about how to maximise health outcome given the resources available. One example might be a comparison of histamine H_2-receptor antagonists (H_2RAs) and H^+/K^+-ATPase (or proton pump) inhibitors (PPIs) for healing reflux oesophagitis. An appropriate CEA might be specified with an outcome measure such as symptom-free days with the success and rates of healing being different for each therapy.

In practice, evidence around the benefits of alternative treatments is derived from clinical trials, systematic reviews and meta-analyses (as described earlier) and estimates of resource use are normally recorded within trials and costed according to national rates (e.g. NHS reference costs, drug tariff). The total costs and benefits associated with each treatment are then compared incrementally. Assuming that PPIs are both more effective and more expensive than H_2RAs, the incremental cost-effectiveness ratio is calculated as follows:

$$\text{Incremental cost-effectiveness ratio} = \frac{\text{Cost of PPI} - \text{Cost of } H_2\text{RA}}{\text{Benefits of PPI} - \text{Benefits of } H_2\text{RA}}$$

If the incremental cost-effectiveness ratio exceeds the value that a payer places on an additional day free of symptoms, then PPIs would not be considered to be cost-effective. However, determining this value requires that a judgement is made by the payer, or that information is available on the least efficient intervention currently in use.

One of the main limitations of CEA is its inability to compare medicines with other health technologies that produce health improvement in different, or in more than one dimension. For this reason, health economists prefer to use cost-utility analyses.

Cost-utility analysis

Cost-utility analyses (CUAs) are appropriate when the health effects of two or more alternatives can be measured in terms of their overall impact on quantity and quality of life – the two most important patient-related out-come measures. They are a special form of CEA, in which the consequences are measured in terms of quality-adjusted life-years (QALYs). QALYs are calculated by estimating the total life-years gained from a treatment and weighing each year (or part thereof) with a quality-of-life ('utility') score. The utility value is 0 for 'dead' and 1 for 'full health'. Various methods, including the EQ-5D questionnaire, can be used to quantify health-related quality of life, to provide a single summary score (see Page 52).

The advantage of the QALY is that it incorporates quality and quantity of life in a common currency that allows comparison of interventions from different clinical areas. QALYs can therefore address issues of allocative efficiency. Allocative efficiency answers questions about achieving the right mixture of healthcare programmes to maximise the health of society. It may be used to compare very different interventions, such as chemotherapy in advanced breast cancer, surgery for coronary artery bypass grafting and medicines for diabetes. For this reason, CUAs are the preferred form of economic evaluation in appraisals by NICE and other health technology appraisal agencies.

Economic analysis

Clinical trials generally do not capture all the data required for an economic analysis. Moreover, it is often appropriate to project the results of clinical trials beyond the time horizon of analysis, to capture predicted lifetime costs and benefits. Economic analyses are essentially mathematical models used to compile data from various sources and to test the robustness of underlying assumptions and uncertainties. The most common forms of economic models are decision analyses (represented schematically as decision trees) and Markov models, which are helpful for modelling the progression of chronic diseases. Within a Markov model, a disease is divided into health states (e.g. remission, progression, death), and during a chosen period of time each individual is given a probability of moving from one state to another. Estimates of the use of resources and health effects are also attached to each state. The model is then cycled to produce long term estimates of cost-effectiveness in hypothetical defined patient cohorts.

Judging whether any medicine represents good value for money (and whether it will therefore be recommended for use by a decision making body) depends on whether the incremental cost-effectiveness ratio falls within an acceptable range. NICE considers that health care interventions that cost less than £20 000–30 000 per QALY gained are cost-effective. There are also special dispensations for appraising end-of-life treatments for rare conditions, accepting that the NHS may be prepared to spend more per QALY in such cases. In practice, consideration must also be given to affordability. An intervention that gained one extra year of life at an additional cost of £10 000 might be thought highly cost-effective, but if five million people merited treatment it might not be affordable. Some health technology appraisal organisations (such as the All Wales Medicines Strategy Group) make explicit consideration of affordability, while others (such as NICE) do not.

Critical appraisal of economic evaluations

As with clinical evidence, there is also variable quality in the conduct and reporting of economic evaluations. There are many potential sources of bias, particularly when data are modelled. Again a checklist, for use in appraising an economic evaluation, such as the one provided in Box 7.2, is valuable.

Box 7.2 *Checklist for the critical appraisal of economic evaluations*[14]

1   Was a well-defined question posed in answerable form?
   - Did the study examine both costs and effects of the medicine?
   - Did the study involve a comparison of alternatives?
   - Was a perspective of the analysis stated and was the study placed in a particular decision-making context?
2   Was a comprehensive description of alternatives given?
   - Can you tell who did what to whom, where and how often?
3   Was there evidence that effectiveness had been established?
   - Was this done through a randomised, controlled clinical trial?
   - Did the trial reflect what would happen in regular practice?
   - Was effectiveness established through an overview of clinical studies?
   - Were observational data or assumptions used to establish effectiveness? If so, what are the potential biases in results?
4   Were all the important and relevant costs and consequences for each alternative identified?
   - Was the range wide enough for the research question at hand?

(continued overleaf)

- Did it cover all relevant perspectives (e.g. social, patients and third-party payers)?
- Were capital costs and operating costs included?

5 Were costs and consequences measured accurately/appropriately?
- Were any of the identified items omitted from measurement?
- Were there any special circumstances (e.g. joint use of resources) that made measurement difficult?

6 Were costs and consequences valued credibly?
- Were the sources of all values clearly identified (e.g. market values, patient preferences)?
- Were market values employed for changes involving resources gained or depleted?
- Where market values were absent (e.g. volunteer labour) or market values did not reflect values, were adjustments made to approximate market values?
- Was the valuation of consequences appropriate for the question posed (i.e. appropriate type of analysis (cost-minimisation analysis, cost-effectiveness analysis, cost-utility analysis) selected?)

7 Were costs and consequences adjusted for differential timing?
- Were costs and consequences which occur in the future discounted to their present values?
- Was any justification given for the discount rate used?

8 Was an incremental analysis performed?
- Were the additional (incremental) costs generated by one alternative over another compared with the additional effects, benefits, or utilities generated?

9 Was allowance made for uncertainty?
- Were appropriate sensitivity analyses performed?
- If a sensitivity analysis was done, was justification provided for the range of values for study parameters?
- Were study results sensitive to changes in the values?

10 Did presentation/discussion of results include all issues of concern?
- Were the conclusions based on a ratio of costs to consequences?
- Were results compared with other studies?
- Was the generalisability of the study discussed?
- Were other important factors considered, e.g. ethics?
- Did the study discuss implementation issues?

Reproduced with permission from Oxford University Press.[14]

The NHS Economic Evaluation Database (www.crd.york.ac.uk) catalogues published economic evaluations, includes a summary of the key findings and a critique of the methods employed.

Evidence-based pharmacy practice

Novel pharmaceutical services should be subject to the same level of evidential standards as novel pharmaceutical technologies, such as medicines. The same hierarchy of evidence applies to services and other interventions, thus one of the most valuable forms of evidence is meta-analysis of RCTs. Outcome measures used in studies of pharmacy services should ideally be patient-related outcome measures, rather than disease oriented. Similarly the terms used to show treatment effects for medicines should be used in pharmacy practice as should the same statistical rigour. Few studies of pharmacy services incorporate economic evaluations, but increasingly these are important for demonstrating the potential costs and benefits of novel services. Systematic reviews are becoming available for a number of pharmacy interventions and much of the work done to date is covered in Chapters 11–14 of this book.

References

1. Cochrane A. *Effectiveness and Efficiency: Random reflections on health services*. London: Royal Society of Medicine Press, 1999.
2. Sackett DL, Rosenberg WM, Gray JA *et al*. Evidence based medicine: what it is and what it isn't. *BMJ* 1996; 312: 71–72.
3. CRASH trial collaborators. Effect of intravenous corticosteroids on death within 14 days in 10008 adults with clinically significant head injury (MRC CRASH trial): a randomised placebo-controlled trial. *Lancet* 2004; 364: 1321–1328.
4. Lau J, Antman EM, Jimenez-Silva J *et al*. Cumulative meta-analysis of therapeutic trials for myocardial infarction. *N Engl J Med* 1992; 327(4): 248–254.
5. Sackett DL, Straus SE, Richardson WS *et al*. *Evidence-Based Medicine: How to practice and teach EBM*, 2nd ed. Edinburgh: Churchill Livingstone, 2000.
6. Echt DS, Liebson PR, Mitchell LB *et al*. Mortality and morbidity in patients receiving encainide, flecainide, or placebo: the Cardiac Arrhythmia Suppression Trial. *N Engl J Med* 1991; 324: 781–788.
7. Riggs BL, Hodgson SF, O'Fallon WM *et al*. Effect of fluoride treatment on the fracture rate in postmenopausal women with osteoporosis. *N Engl J Med* 1990; 322: 802–809.
8. Moher D, Schulz KF, Altman D. The CONSORT statement: revised recommendations for improving the quality of reports of parallel-group randomized trials. *JAMA* 2001; 285: 1987–1991.
9. Jüni P, Altman DG, Egger M. Systematic reviews in health care: assessing the quality of controlled clinical trials. *BMJ* 2001; 323(7303): 42–46.
10. Schulz KF, Chalmers I, Hayes RJ *et al*. Empirical evidence of bias: dimensions of methodological quality associated with estimates of treatment effects in controlled trials. *JAMA* 1995; 273(5): 408–412.
11. Sheldon TA, Cullum N, Dawson D *et al*. What's the evidence that NICE guidance has been implemented? Results from a national evaluation using time series analysis, audit of patient notes and interviews. *BMJ* 2004; 329: 999–1004.

12. The NHS Information Centre, Prescribing Support Unit. *Use of NICE Appraised Medicines in the NHS in England – Experimental Statistics*, 2009.

13. McGlynn EA, Asch SM, Adams J *et al.* The quality of health care delivered to adults in the United States. *New Engl J Med* 2003; 348: 2635–2645.

14. Drummond MF, Sculpher MJ, Torrance GW *et al. Methods for the Economic Evaluation of Health Care Programmes*, 3rd edn. Oxford: Oxford University Press, 2005.

8

Working together

Fiona Harris

The aim of this chapter is to give a brief overview of multi-disciplinary and multi-agency working. Multi-disciplinary working within health is generally taken to mean people from more than one discipline working together, such as doctors, pharmacists and nurses. Multi-agency working is wider than this and involves people from different agencies working together, such as health services and local councils. Local government (councils) has responsibility for sevices such as social care, education, environmental health and leisure. These services can impact on the health of the local population, for example social care workers, who provide services such as personal care, advice and support to vulnerable families, frail elderly and children. Other organisations may include police and fire services or non-statutory organisations such as the voluntary sector. Voluntary organisations, such as charities and church groups, also provide a great many services that impact on health; therefore it is important to involve them in working together with health-related organisations.

Working together with other disciplines and other agencies is increasingly important to pharmacists and pharmaceutical services in all sectors. Within the UK, the term 'partnership working' is now used more commonly for all types of working together, but there is nothing new about partnership working. As discussed in Chapter 2, the wider determinants of health include education, crime, housing and the environment; therefore no single agency alone can succeed in improving the health of a particular population. However, in recent years partnership working has become more of an imperative. It is safe to say that of recent policy documents from central government have consistently advocated working in partnership.

In 1998 the DoH published a document *Partnership in Action*[1] in which it advocated that 'The strategic agenda is to work across boundaries ... underpinned by a duty of partnership .... Past efforts to tackle these problems have shown that concentrating on single elements of the way services work together ... without looking at the system as a whole does not work.' In more recent policy documents,[2] legal duties have been established to ensure that statutory organisations such as local government, NHS bodies, police and fire services work together with non-statutory organisations such as voluntary groups. Partnership has therefore not only become a legal, but almost a moral, imperative.

In Scotland, Community Health Partnerships, established in 2004 and which effectively replaced PCTs, were specifically aimed at ensuring that health services and other relevant local government services could increase their joint working. In England, many PCTs now have specialists in partnership working (often based within the public health directorate), whose role is to develop and sustain partnerships. Indeed the expectation that the Director of Public Health has a joint role encompassing both health and government both at regional level and in many PCTs illustrates the importance placed on partnerships within public health practice (see Chapter 1).

Partnership working

Health and social care are complex systems, yet people with complex health needs frequently need input from a multitude of different professionals in both sectors. It is important to appreciate that different parts of health and social care agencies are interdependent, so that action by one agency will have unintended consequences for other agencies and for the system as a whole. A good example of this is the issue around discharge from hospital. In the mid to late 90s, social services often delayed developing care packages or identifying a place in a residential or nursing home for patients who had been treated in hospital. As long as patients were in hospital, their care was being funded by the NHS, at no cost to social services. The consequence of this was a reduction in available beds for patients with acute health needs (so called bed-blocking). Another impact of this delay on patients was an increasing risk of institutionalisation resulting in an inability to return home. More recently the drive for the NHS to reduce hospital stays, increase bed availability and increase throughput of patients has resulted in the converse situation. Patients may be discharged earlier with more complex needs, therefore the care packages required are more complex and more costly to social services.[3]

In the UK, there has been considerable fragmentation of the health service over the past 15 years, owing to devolution, which created four different NHS organisations, and the large number of policy changes. While differences inevitably occur between the home countries, most of the principles outlined here apply throughout the UK.

One important result of the fragmentation of health services is that a variety of different organisations provide care to the same population, for example, PCTs, community services, acute trusts and mental health trusts, which could result in duplication of service provision. A disease-oriented approach to healthcare provision can have the effect of duplicating effort both at an organisational level (within health and social care) and at an individual patient level, where a patient with more than one condition may be receiving services from multiple disciplines and agencies. Furthermore, the drive to attain specific targets or reduce costs within one organisation can have adverse impacts on another. Partnership working has the potential to reduce these issues. An example is the Partnerships for Older People Projects (POPP) which was launched in 2005 to develop and evaluate services and approaches for older people aimed at promoting health, well-being and independence and preventing or delaying the need for higher intensity or institutional care. The focus of the POPP programme has been to test and evaluate different models of service through 29 local authority-led pilots. The pilots have aimed to create a sustainable shift in resources and culture away from institutional and hospital-based crisis care for older people towards earlier, targeted interventions for older people within their own homes and communities.[4]

Fragmentation and lack of continuity of services is not just a problem for the UK. Different organisations provide acute and long term care in many countries. There are a number of examples of 'integrated care' (another term for partnership working) within the USA. For example, an initiative which provides fully integrated health and long term care for community dwelling elderly people, who are eligible for nursing home care, has been shown to reduce hospital admission.[5]

There are major challenges in bringing together health and social services to provide a more joined-up and holistic approach to people with multiple needs, whether these be frail older people, people with mental health problems, people with learning difficulties, or people with long term conditions such as heart failure or chronic obstructive pulmonary disease. This is the case, irrespective of how different systems work. There are even greater challenges in trying to coordinate and implement health improvement programmes between multiple agencies such as those designed to help in reducing smoking, supporting people to achieve a healthy weight and tackling the harm caused by the misuse of alcohol. This is mainly due to the confused picture in terms of organisational responsibility for leading on prevention.

The key barriers to partnership working include[6]:

- structural divisions – for example, NHS for healthcare versus local authority for social care
- separate legal and financial frameworks – health and social care are controlled mainly by very different sets of primary and secondary legislation, although some legislation covers both

- distinct organisational and professional cultures – not only are social and healthcare generally provided by different organisations but within health there are different organisations, providing care such as independent contractors including community pharmacists, hospitals and community services
- governance and accountability differences – for example, in England the NHS is directly responsible to the national government through the Secretary of State, whereas social care is responsible to local government and locally elected politicians.

However, to deal with the complexity of the health and social problems that we face, and to respond to changing demographics, increasing costs of health and social care and higher expectations of patients, multi-agency responses are necessary.

Defining partnerships

Glasby and Dickinson provide a useful summary of the recent discourse on partnership working.[6] While the term is extensively used in policy documents, partnership working has not been clearly defined and often means different things to different people in different contexts. In addition, UK health-related policies use the term partnership in several contexts, while some other ways of working together are not termed partnership at all. For example:

- Public–private partnerships are partnerships between the public and private sectors designed to deliver services and infrastructure, including health services. These are contractual and legally binding partnerships, the most common of which is the private finance initiative.
- All areas in England are expected to have local strategic partnerships, set up by local government. These are designed to bring together different groups within the public and private sectors, businesses and other groups to help in implementing community strategies and local area agreements. In contrast to public–private partnerships, local strategic partnerships are non-statutory but are driven by central government guidance and seek to help achieve national targets.
- The NHS Act 2006 established 'Section 75 agreements', which enable the pooling of resources between the NHS and health-related local authority services, to improve the joining-up of services. This legally allows one agency to commission services on behalf of another. For instance the NHS can commission certain mental health services on behalf of the local authority or vice versa.

Other terms used for working together include collaboration, joint working and a whole systems approach. The extent to which organisations can work together varies from simple sharing of information (which is often far from simple especially where it involves individual data), through coordinating activities to formal partnerships. Managed clinical networks are another way of describing multi-agency working which seeks to enhance patient care.

The general consensus (adapted from reference 3) is that partnership working:

- involves negotiation between people from different agencies who are committed to working together for a specific purpose in an ongoing relationship
- should provide benefit to individuals (service users/patients) that could not have been provided by any single agency acting alone – the added value
- should have shared goals and agreed ways of achieving those goals through formal expression of purpose and plan to implement – the 'win–win' situation.

Partners within a partnership retain the right of exit at any time, which differs from a contractual arrangement which is legally binding. Partnership working usually requires aligning resources or even pooling resources and this is often where tensions start to build. Partnerships are relationships and relationships are inevitably about power and control, but they are also to do with dialogue, negotiation, and the development of shared objectives and involve real people in real situations, which mean they will be influenced by individuals' personalities.[7]

Advantages of partnership working

The Audit Commission in 1998[8] suggested the five main reasons to work in partnership were to:

- coordinate packages of care
- tackle the 'wicked' issues (that is, very difficult problems we really don't know how to tackle)
- reduce the impact of organisational fragmentation
- meet statutory requirements
- bid to gain access to new resources that could only be accessed by a range of partners working together. An example of this is funding to establish health action zones or more recently, local area agreements.

This was supported by Payne[6,9] who highlighted six reasons for multi-professional working:

- bringing together skills
- sharing information
- continuity of care
- apportioning responsibility and accountability
- coordination in planning
- coordination in delivering resources for the benefit of users.

Evidence for partnership working

While the benefits or positive aspects of partnership working are frequently emphasised, there is very little evidence to support these advantages. 'No evidence of effect' is not however, the same as 'evidence of no effect'. While the former may be true for partnership working, there is also considerable evidence of the impact of failure to work in partnership. Much of what has been evaluated and published to date has focused on processes and the impact on organisations. Two systematic reviews identified that there is evidence on perceptions of success, which are important, but that benefits in terms of outcomes for users, providers and commissioners was very basic. Indeed the acid test for a partnership is the experience of people using services, i.e. that they achieve good outcomes.

As the DoH pointed out in 1998,[1] it is where partnerships don't exist, and sterile arguments around the artificial boundaries of organisations persist that vulnerable people fall through the gaps and harm may be caused. To address this, the Care Quality Commission was established in 2009, as an independent regulator which aims to make sure better care is provided by hospitals, care homes and community services and champions joined-up services across health and social care settings in England. The Commission's findings are important for health professionals everywhere. A report published by the Commission following the high profile death of a young child, indicated poor communication between health professionals and across agencies, plus lack of clear roles and responsibilities within some health organisations.[10] In relation to pharmacists, the commission has identified that there is inadequate sharing of information about medicines between secondary and primary care and vice versa in many areas of England.[11] It is likely that similar problems occur in many countries.

To make partnerships work a better understanding of what motivates 'real people' to work together, the context in which they operate and potential benefits in terms of outcomes for service users is required. Increasing limitations in the availability of resources within the public sector including both health and social care has recently given new impetus to the need to improve this understanding.[7] There is a need to achieve more with less resources and partnership working has the potential to minimise duplication of effort, as well as preventing unnecessary use of resources.

Making partnerships work

There are increasing numbers of tools and frameworks available that are designed to support partnership working. These can form very useful checklists, although they may over-simplify the challenges within partnerships.[6] A widely used framework is the Partnership Assessment Tool developed by the

University of Leeds.[6,12] This tool is based on six partnership principles and allows local partnerships to assess their achievement against the principles. The key principles are to:

- recognise and accept the need for partnership
- develop clarity and realism of purpose
- ensure commitment and ownership
- develop and maintain trust
- create clear and robust partnership arrangements
- monitor, measure and learn.

Another useful tool is the Working Partnership developed by the Health Development Agency (now part of NICE).[6,13] The Working Partnership is a more in-depth tool that focuses on the key elements of good practice:

- leadership (shared vision, ownership and commitment)
- organisation (transparent management, flexible working, communication and public participation)
- strategy (strategic development, information, evaluation, action and review)
- learning (valuing people, developing knowledge and skills and supporting innovation)
- resources (pooling resources, using information and technology appropriately)
- programmes (developing coordinated programmes and integrated services through joint planning, focused delivery and monitoring and reviewing progress).

Although these tools are necessarily simplistic they do provide a useful self-assessment and can make sense of some of the barriers that exist within partnerships.

Partnerships must be worked at if they are going to succeed. All those working within a partnership must recognise the fact that each may have the same ultimate goal but the means of achieving those goals may be very different. An example of a partnership approach is that of tackling the harm caused by alcohol misuse. The use of alcohol has a significant impact on health (see Chapter 2) with alcohol misuse being the second biggest cause of preventable deaths in developed world. However, alcohol impacts on a range of local government and other agencies, besides health (Box 8.1).

England's national alcohol strategy *Safe, Sensible, Social*[14] identifies what needs to be done on a local basis (Figure 8.1). The individual partners involved in this strategy will have very different approaches to achieving their goals. While all agencies are interested in preventing the immediate problems they face and reducing their costs, their approach and drivers maybe very different.

Box 8.1 *The impact of alcohol use on various agencies. Adapted from reference 14*

Health

- Immediate treatment (accident and emergency/emergency admissions/ambulance)
- Long term treatment to reduce addictive behaviours (specialist services)
- Long term treatment of liver conditions/cancers of the upper gastrointestinal tract and other associated illness

Police

- Policing night-time economy
- Anti social behaviour/drink driving/assaults
- Criminal justice
- Domestic violence

Social care/children's services

- Support for patients with health and social care needs
- Support for families affected by domestic violence
- Safe-guarding (children and adults)
- Teenage pregnancy

Licensing/planning

- Night-time economy
- Regulation/underage sales
- Litter/waste

General costs for England estimated to be £20 billion

- NHS: £3 billion
- Criminal justice system: £10 billion
- UK industry: £7 billion

In England

- 8 million drink twice the weekly recommended limits
- 2 million drink over twice the recommended weekly limits
- 1.4 million drink more than twice the recommended daily limit in a single session

Alcohol-related harm has increased significantly in the past decade

- In England, hospitalisation rates almost doubled between 2002/3 and 2007/8

At a local level, with an average population of 200 000, costs could be £63 million.

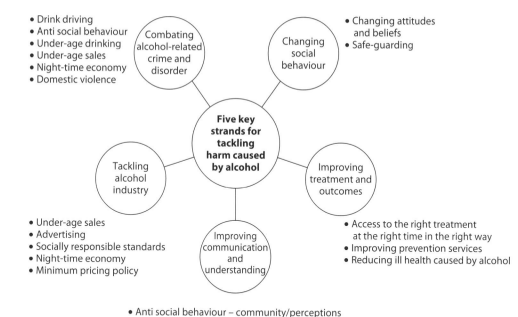

Figure 8.1 Tackling harm caused by alcohol. Adapted from reference 14.

The key tensions exist between the police, health and the local authority. In trying to reduce excessive consumption of alcohol and therefore the harm caused, the police and health have similar goals. On the other hand, the local authority also has a goal of developing the local economy to encourage business, jobs and local investment which can include the night-time economy. Interestingly there will be an internal tension within the local authority between the departments focusing on economic development and environmental health which has the responsibility of keeping the streets clean. To achieve the partnership goal of reducing harm from alcohol, a 'win–win' solution must be found – this is where innovation and lateral thinking can be beneficial. Achieving a 'win–win' often needs some sort of compromise and action requires sharing of resources, which can create additional tension in a climate of tight public spending.

Partnership working and pharmacy

Access to quality healthcare through good clinical practice has increasingly been recognised as a significant determinant of health, in the UK and elsewhere. This includes the use of pharmaceutical interventions. UK government policy has focused on standardising clinical decision making, particularly with pharmaceutical interventions, to improve clinical practice, although different mechanisms exist in the different home countries (see Chapters 7 and 14). An important public health task for pharmacists in whatever setting they work is to support patients to take their medicines appropriately, to maximise the benefit of the intervention.[15] This being the case, it could be argued that pharmacists have to work in partnership with patients and their carers, with GPs, with community services and with social care, as well as working across the 'boundary' between primary and secondary care. Effective use of medicines is central to the patient experience and to the quality of healthcare.

Medication is the most common form of medical intervention in the UK, yet various studies have found that up to 50% of medicines are not taken as prescribed[16] and adverse reactions to medicines are implicated in 5–17% of hospital admissions.[17] Reduced compliance and failure to achieve concordance with prescribed medicines-taking can prevent full benefits from being obtained and cause unnecessary ill health, premature death and significant avoidable cost to the NHS.[18] Many problems with medicines could be prevented by monitoring the effects of long term drug therapy, by identifying those at risk and by modifying their medication where necessary.[19] In terms of preventing hospital admissions and harm to individuals, working in partnership to help people manage their medicines is crucial. A case study illustrating partnership working involving pharmacists is shown in Box 8.2.

Key aspects of partnership working illustrated by this are:

- training key workers in intermediate care on how to use the COUNT® tool to ensure a consistent approach to identifying a medicine-related problem
- the professional relationship between primary care pharmacists and GPs, which provided access to medical records and also ensured that pharmacists' views were respected and taken into account when reviewing patient's medication
- detailed discussion with the patient, carer and/or wider family in the patient's own home to consider practical solutions to medicine-related problems
- a post-visit discussion with all appropriate healthcare professionals to inform them of the findings, ensuring agreement and continuity of care.

In summary, it is fair to say that partnership working in its broadest sense is important, possibly vital. To achieve good health outcomes, professionals working in both health and social services cannot work in isolation. Although at the moment we don't have a solid evidence base to prove this, nor is there a really concrete framework to ensure success, we do know what happens when partnership working fails. In the short term, in lieu of the requisite evidence, the key is that any partners working together need to be clear about what they are trying to achieve and build in monitoring and

Box 8.2 *A case study of pharmacists working in partnership*

In Guildford and Waverley (now part of Surrey Primary Care Trust), the population has a greater proportion of people aged over 85 than England as a whole and also significant pockets of deprivation, particularly in barriers to accessing services, because the area is relatively rural. The aging population has a high prevalence of chronic disease and consequently high medicines use. The trust set up an intermediate care service, involving both health and social care workers, to prevent potential admissions to secondary care and provide additional support to recently discharged patients. The service identified that a significant number of patients had problems managing their medicines, which was perceived as creating a major workload for them.

To address this and to maximise the benefits and minimise the risks of medicines by ensuring that patients understand and are happy with prescribed treatments, a training package was developed to enable non-clinical, intermediate care, key workers to recognise potential medicine-related problems. This was based on a mnemonic, COUNT®.

- Confused over what the medicine is for and how and when to take it.
- Over-ordering medicine – stockpiling, sharing, overuse, underuse.
- Unable to open packaging – unable to unscrew the lids on bottles or open foil packs or use inhalers (agility).
- Not taking medicine – forgetting, or choosing not to take medicine.
- Too many or too few journeys – collecting medicines every week and access issues.

For patients identified with medicine-related problems, the relevant primary care pharmacist then reviewed their medicines with them at home, in conjunction with their GP, using medical records. A clear case definition was developed to ensure that patients most at risk were targeted, while managing the caseload within existing trust pharmacy resources. To evaluate this, pharmacists assessed the likely impact of not having intervened, using a standard risk assessment tool commonly used to assess potential hospital avoidance, and GP views were obtained by interview. The risk assessment results indicated that the pharmacist input reduced hospital admissions, and reviews of patients' records indicated a reduction in medicines waste, as well as improving communication and understanding between the intermediate care team, general practice and pharmacists.

evaluation to ensure the outcomes that are important to service users are achieved. More importantly, pharmacists, along with other health professionals should actively seek out and welcome opportunities for partnership working, since this should result in the ultimate goal of greater patient benefit, even though demonstrating this may be difficult. Helping to improve sharing of information between primary and secondary care, as advocated by the Care Quality Commission, would be a good place to start.

References

1. Department of Health. *Partnership in Action*. London: Department of Health, 1998.
2. Department of Health. *Our Health, Our Care, Our Say*. London: Department of Health 2006.
3. Plamping D, Gordon P, Pratt J. Modernising the NHS: practical partnerships for health and local authorities. *BMJ* 2000; 320: 1723–1725.
4. Details on POPPs can be found on http://www.dhcarenetworks.org.uk/Prevention/POPPs.
5. Kodner D. Integrated service models. In: Glasby J, Dickinson H, eds. *International Perspectives on Heath and Social care: Partnership working in action*. Chichester: Wiley-Blackwell, 2008.
6. Glasby J, Dickinson H. *Partnership Working in Health and Social Care*. Policy Press 2008.
7. Popay J, Williams G. Partnership in health: beyond the rhetoric. *J Epidemiol Commun Health* 1998; 52: 410–411.
8. Audit Commission. *A Fruitful Partnership: Effective partnership working*. Audit Commission, 1998.
9. Payne M. *Teamwork in Multi-professional Care*. Basingstoke: Palgrave Macmillan, 2000.
10. Care Quality Commission. *Review Of the Involvement and Action Taken by Health Bodies in Relation to the Death of Baby P*. London: Care Quality Commission, 2009.
11. Care Quality Commission. *Managing Patients' Medicines After Discharge from Hospital*. London: Care Quality Commission, 2009.
12. Hardy B, Hudson B, Waddington E. *Assessing Strategic Partnership: The Partnership Assessment Tool*, London: Nuffield Institute for Health, 2003.
13. Markwell S, Watson J, Speller V *et al. The Working Partnership*. London: Health Development Agency, 2003. http://www.nice.org.uk/niceMedia/documents/working_partnership_1.pdf
14. Department of Health. *Safe Sensible Social*. London: Department of Health, 2007.
15. Hicks N. In: Griffiths S, Hunter DJ, eds. *Perspectives in Public Health*. Oxford: Radcliffe Medical Press, 1999: 223–234.
16. Royal Pharmaceutical Society of Great Britain. *From Compliance to Concordance*. London: RPSGB, 1997.
17. Department of Health. *Medicines and Older People* (supplement to the NSF for Older People), London: Department of Health, 2001.
18. Royal College of Physicians. Medicines for older people. *J R Coll Physicians* 1997; 31: 254–257.
19. MeRec Bulletin. *Prescribing for the Older Person,* MeReC, 2000, 11: 10.

9

Developing pharmacy services

David Pfleger

The health needs of populations and the health policy context within which pharmacy services are delivered are not static. Pharmacists therefore need to develop new and modify the existing services they provide in response to changes in health policy and the needs of the population they serve. Service development is therefore relevant to all practising pharmacists. In the UK, both NHS and privately funded services, i.e. purchased by the client or an organisation on their behalf, may be developed by community pharmacists. If an NHS-funded service, such development proposals will need to be scrutinised and accepted by the local PCT or health board.

Pharmacists working in hospitals may want to develop a new service, but have to convince managers of its value and a service proposal is a useful tool in doing this. Hence a service proposal must be drafted and put to the relevant body or individuals, for them to consider whether they will commission, or authorise, the service or not. Wherever pharmacists work, whether the local health system is mainly nationally or locally commissioned, it is likely that there will be opportunities for some degree of local commissioning or development of services.

Service development proposals

This section explains how a service proposal should be written or critiqued. It should be of use to pharmacists making the case to a manager within an organisation about developing a service, those trying to gain resources from a healthcare organisation to put in place a pharmacy service locally or for those who are reviewing a proposal for service development from the commissioning perspective.

Service development proposals set out a plan for a new or revised service. Pharmacists may be involved in developing new services in any area of health need, such as substance misuse, diabetes, older people on multiple medicines.

In general, development proposals explain the need for the service and describe the evidence for the model of care the service aims to provide, both in terms of financial and clinical outcomes, along with details of how the service will be run and evaluated. Service developments are more likely to be successful if they are:

- based on need
- fulfilling the drivers of the purchaser, e.g. local or national priorities
- delivering quantifiable health gain or improved service, e.g. improved access, improved clinical outcomes
- evidence based
- cost-effective
- supported by robust clinical governance structures
- designed to 'fit' with and complement other existing/planned services.

Before starting a proposal

Once you have an initial idea for the service you want to develop, it is useful to think about which key stakeholders will need to be involved in developing the proposal and taking it through to a commissioning decision. Developing a service proposal without the input of commissioners and users is likely to end in failure. It is important not to end up with a fully worked up proposal, only to find it doesn't fit with the local commissioning plan, that the timing of the proposal has just missed the finance window in the commissioning cycle or that there is already a plan in place for a service to be offered by another healthcare provider. Therefore it is useful to start the development with a scoping exercise. This involves summarising what you are aiming to do and most importantly, identifying how it fits with the local healthcare organisation's priorities and work plans. It allows you to begin quantifying the work that will be needed to develop the full proposal and identify the key people and organisations that you will need to involve. It may be that pharmacy does not need to take the lead role. The service proposed may involve only a supporting role for pharmacy or may be part of a much wider service involving other providers as well.

Identify the potential stakeholders

A stakeholder is a person, group of people or organisation which could be affected by or could affect your proposed service. They can be individuals or groups from within your organisation or other healthcare organisations or agencies who are either involved in using or delivering the service. Some may have the potential to block your proposal at any stage of the commissioning process. It is important to identify at which level or stage of development particular stakeholders either hold influence or are needed as part of the proposal development.[1]

Stakeholders are likely to include pharmacists, managers, people with responsibility for taking the lead on the area targeted by your service, other clinical staff (GPs, nurses, other health professionals), patients and clients and the public. Local professional advisory groups, such as the local medical committee could also be regarded as stakeholders. Finding out who the variety of stakeholders and stakeholder groups are may require some initial discussions, but is important, because it will potentially smooth the path of service development.

Identify a steering group

It is useful to have a steering group to strategically manage the development of the proposal and also to act as a sounding board for the various drafts of the proposal as it is developed. A steering group can be large or small, depending on the size and purpose of the proposal. It offers a wider group of people a stake in the service development and can provide support for the development as it is taken through from initial idea to commissioning. For this reason it is useful to ensure that key stakeholders, including those that have the greatest potential to block your proposal, are involved in the steering group.

Structure and content of the proposal

Where a local commissioning framework already exists there may be specific guidance as to how proposals should be presented. Generally, service development proposals can be split into six key elements, which will be examined in turn:

- local and national policy context
- defining local need
- evidence base for service development
- service specification
- implementation and evaluation
- business case.

In addition a proposal will need an executive summary, references and possibly appendices.

Local and national policy context

This section of the proposal should set the scene and demonstrate the evidence base for the proposed service. Chapters 11–13 illustrate the evidence for services which have been developed and Chapter 7 lists some other possible sources of evidence. Since any new pharmacy service must be designed to meet a health need and fit with relevant policy if it is to be viable, the background to the need and the policy must be explained. This may start by describing relevant health and/or social policy at a national level, providing a summary of the current policy direction for pharmacy and pharmacy services.

It is important to remember that a number of people will be reading a proposal. Some will be pharmacists, but others may include a finance director or lay member of the health organisation's managing board. Therefore it should not be assumed that readers will be familiar with pharmacy or the health policy/background for the area the proposal covers. It is very important to link national need/policy to the local situation. Information about this can be obtained from, for example, the annual report of the local Director of Public Health (see Chapter 1), local health plans, JSNAs (see Chapter 6), local pharmacy strategies and so on. As part of this, it is helpful to provide the context within which the service development will take place, by providing a description of the existing local services that the new service will operate alongside or within. For example, a proposal for a sexual health service should provide some information about local sexual health services. In providing the background and introduction, the points in Box 9.1 should be considered.

Box 9.1 *Points to consider in summarising the background to a service development proposal*

- What drivers are shaping policy and service delivery in the area?
- Which policy documents provide the context for pharmacy, the service and the environment in which the service will operate?
- What are the national trends in prevalence and incidence of the condition the proposal targets?
- Are there any relevant clinical standards or descriptors of best practice?
- How does the service development fit with national priorities?
- Is there a local strategy for service development in this area?
- Is a national strategy in place or being developed, which includes pharmacy?
- Does the proposed service fit with local healthcare priorities identified in the Director of Public Health report?
- How will the proposed service contribute to national and local health priorities and targets?
- What, potentially, does pharmacy have to offer? Any unique selling points?

Defining local need

Any proposal must describe the local need for the service (see Chapter 6). Need must be considered in broad terms and not just describe people who may use a pharmacy service. Unless undertaking a fully resourced needs assessment as part of the healthcare organisation's work plan, or responding to one that has already been undertaken, it is likely that this section will rely heavily on an epidemiological approach, backed up by information extracted from local policy documents and reports and from discussions with local experts. It is important when presenting a needs assessment to support a new service development, to be very clear about the aim and scope of the assessment and the approach and methods used. Even if a previous needs assessment is available, information may become out of date quite quickly both in terms of population health indices and the existing local service provision. Frequently within service development proposals, there is more emphasis on demand rather than need and, within pharmacy, considerations of what the pharmacy profession feels is appropriate or would like to do, rather than what is needed.

If there is already existing service provision in place, it is particularly important not just to describe that provision but to describe and evaluate the extent to which that service meets local needs. This then allows the case to be made for the gap or deficiency in service provision that a service development proposal will fill. In providing the evidence of need, the points in Box 9.2

Box 9.2 *Points to consider in identifying need within a service development proposal*

- Has there already been a needs assessment relating to the topic area published locally, elsewhere or in the literature? If so, is it relevant and up to date?
- What epidemiological data are available locally to help assess need?
- Can the need be described in terms of demographic characteristics of those in need and their location? Can the size of the need be estimated?
- Can the likely uptake of the service be estimated, supported by literature or experience elsewhere?
- If local data are not available, what national or otherwise published data can help?
- What services are currently provided locally?
- Are there any reports from stakeholders, e.g. clinicians and patients indicating dissatisfaction with the current services available or expressing need for additional/alternative services?
- What outcomes is the current service producing? Are these outcomes contributing sufficiently to the local healthcare organisation's health improvement targets?
- Are there any particular target groups that do less well or don't engage with existing services?

should be considered. Failure to explain what a new service offers in comparison to existing services may mean the commissioners decide it is not required at all.

Demonstrating the evidence base to support the proposal

Although EBM is well developed, it focuses mainly on interventions directed at the patient. There is also a need to ensure that all service developments are supported by or contribute to the evidence base.[2] Providing there is a clear need for a service, it is necessary to explain the case for pharmacy being involved in addressing this need. This involves describing the evidence, appraising that evidence and clearly quantifying the potential benefits of the pharmacy service. Thus a systematic review of the literature will be necessary and critical appraisal of the studies identified (see Chapter 7). In doing so, the points in Box 9.3 should be considered. The evidence should then be synthesised into a critical appraisal of the identified studies, emphasising the key aspects of design, potential bias and the relevance and validity of the study results and the author's conclusions, together with a summary and overall conclusion, focusing on how the evidence applies to the proposed service.

Box 9.3 *Points to consider in providing the evidence for a service development proposal*

- What is the aim and related research question(s) that will inform a systematic review of the literature?
- Has a systematic review already been published in the area? How up to date is it?
- If no such review is available, or is out of date, what search strategy, databases and other sources will be used to retrieve relevant evidence?
- What inclusion and exclusion criteria will be applied to any published research? For example, should only randomised controlled trials be included? Will searches include the so-called 'grey literature' and if so how? Will evidence from services delivered in other countries be included?
- What primary research evidence is available that demonstrates the value and efficiency of the proposed service?
- How will the evidence be systematically assessed for quality and generalisability to the proposed service development?

It is quite possible that no research studies have been carried out on the proposed service. In fact there is very little evidence for many pharmacy services, which is a major problem for those wishing to develop their public health role. The evidence for a wide variety of pharmacy services is outlined in Chapters 11–13. As with any other intervention, the ideal evidence comes from meta-analyses of randomised controlled trials, but many studies are simply before-and-after comparisons. If there is no evidence at all, it may be necessary to expand the literature review to gather evidence about similar services delivered by other health professionals or similar (but not identical) services delivered by pharmacy. If this is done, it is important to comment on the generalisability of the data. There is nothing wrong with proposing a service for which there is limited evidence, but a slightly different approach may be needed. This could include three stages: a proof of concept study, followed by a pilot and an evaluation, before larger scale roll out.

Those proposing the service must aim to show that the balance of evidence demonstrates that pharmacy can deliver the service and outcomes described, while commissioners are trying to assess the quality of the case for pharmacy providing that service. Service commissioners must therefore be sure that the evidence supports the investment and will provide the health gains described in the proposal.

Service specification

A specification must outline what the service aims to do and how, who will be involved and how it will be introduced and operated. Important points to consider are listed in Box 9.4. Again, it is important not to assume too much pharmacy knowledge on the part of the reader. The service description should include a very clear statement of the service's aims and objectives. Objectives should be 'SMART', i.e. specific, measurable, achievable, realistic and timely. The aims and objectives must also be attractive to, and fit with the strategy of, the commissioning body. Three types of objectives are required: relating to process, health outcomes and satisfaction.

Objectives related to health outcomes are arguably the most important, but may be most likely to be left out or not clearly defined. As outlined in Chapter 7, health outcomes can be patient related or disease oriented. Many disease-oriented outcomes are used as proxies, because it can be much more difficult to determine patient-related outcomes. For example, one ultimate patient-related objective of a smoking cessation service may be to reduce cardiovascular mortality. This would be very hard to demonstrate because of the timescale required, plus the myriad of other factors and interventions which will impact on such an outcome. A smoking cessation service is still likely to provide benefits to users by helping them to quit smoking and reducing their cardiovascular risk, both of which are measurable. Furthermore, both can be assessed within the lifetime of the service intervention, therefore these proxy outcomes would be acceptable in this instance.

A service description should be very clear and concise and demonstrate how the service links with and adds to other existing services and providers, as well as meeting the needs identified. There may be a contractual component to a new service, which should detail who will hold the contract and any specific requirements this will place on those contracted. These could include requirements for specifically trained personnel or availability of a patient consultation area. Many services provided by community pharmacies incorporate such requirements into the contracts with the PCT or other service commissioning body.

Box 9.4 *Points to consider in writing a specification for a service development proposal*

- What are the aims and objectives of the service?
  - What is the overall aim?
  - What are the key health-related outcomes that the service will provide?
  - What are the process outcomes that are important to delivery of the service from user, provider and commissioner perspectives?
  - What outcomes of client satisfaction (both general and specific to the service) are important to delivery of the service?
- What will the service look like?
  - Will it be in all pharmacies or sites or a selected number?
  - What hours will the service operate? How does this link to the needs of your target group(s)?
  - What geographical spread of coverage will be provided?
  - Is there evidence to support a targeting on a geographical basis?
- How will it be delivered?
  - Detail how the service will operate including any communication that needs to take place, e.g. referrals/updates of patient records and how such things will take place
  - Include relevant protocols or guidelines or refer to how they will be developed if the proposal is successful
- What are the contractual arrangements?
  - Schedule of payments
  - Methodology for payment claims and processing procedures
  - Anti fraud measures
  - Any legal contractual definitions required, e.g. training requirements/continuing professional development requirements

Services can be general, offered by all pharmacies in a locality or may be targeted at specific groups, requiring selected provision, for example, in areas of greatest deprivation. A novel, hospital-based service may be delivered by specialist staff in specific wards, for example, hypertension management in the stroke ward or a general service across all wards and specialties such as a service which aims to improve antibiotic prescribing. Either case requires justification. A service description should also clearly identify and justify whether the service will be provided by pharmacists or well-trained support staff. Good use of skill-mix is an important factor in developing and delivering novel services in pharmacy, given the increasing clinical role of pharmacists.

Service implementation

In drafting a proposal, it is essential to explain how a new service will be implemented, identifying any potential barriers and issues and how these may be managed. In practice, implementation may present more challenges than anticipated, so planning how to do this is vital. A poor implementation phase may damage service development so much that the new service fails to embed quickly enough or may even lead to the service failing.

To succeed, a novel service ideally needs the support of relevant stakeholders before the proposal is sent to the commissioning body. Many novel services within pharmacy fail to do this, instead developing services unilaterally. The importance of ensuring that some of the key stakeholders are engaged through an advisory group or as part of the development team cannot be over-emphasised. Engaging the stakeholders and also harnessing the support of relevant local professional groups such as the local medical committee, local consultant committee or local pharmaceutical committee could be regarded as the first phase of implementation. This can take time and may require the support of a local 'champion', who may be outside pharmacy.

The second phase is the countdown, when the launch date is set. There are likely to be many issues to sort out before a service goes live, including training, marketing, administration and ensuring that payment systems and governance systems are in place. Finally the service requires to be launched. This may involve organising a meeting of relevant practitioners to promote the service, distributing promotional materials, setting up a telephone line or any number of alternative ways of informing people about the service who need to be aware of it. It is important to ensure that sufficient resources are available to troubleshoot any unexpected issues as they arise. It is also important to seek initial feedback during this phase, to ensure the front line practitioners delivering the service have the support they need. Sometimes what worked in a pilot may not translate as expected to a wider service or a pilot may not go as smoothly as you had planned. A list of points to consider in implementation is given in Box 9.5.

Box 9.5 *Points to consider in implementing a service*

- How will the service be implemented?
- Which stakeholders will be engaged and how?
- Will the service need to be piloted? If so, how will it be done?
- How will the pilot be evaluated?
- Will the service require an education and training package to be written, delivered or undertaken? If so, what will be the aims and objectives and how will competence or completion be assessed and recorded/certificated?
- How will you recruit people/pharmacies to deliver the service?
- How will the service be launched?
- How will other professionals who may be affected or expected to use the service be informed about it?
- How will patients or the public be informed, if the service is aimed at them?
- How will problems of unexpectedly high or low demand for the service be dealt with?

Business case

A business case looks at the gains for the resources used and may highlight the risks associated with the proposed development and also those of not going ahead with it. All business cases must have a perspective from which the case is made. For a service development proposal in the vast majority of cases the perspective will be that of the commissioning body.

Resources used in delivering a service include money of course, but also space, equipment and staff. These are all inputs to a service. For a proposal to be successful, the outputs of a novel service should also be identified. These may be the health outcomes identified earlier, but, in the case of independent community pharmacy contractors, where a proposed service is to be privately funded, by the client or end user, there is obviously a need for the service to be profitable. There are many examples of such services which may have an impact on public health, for example, the supply of advice and products within weight management programmes, sale of emergency contraception, privately funded screening for diabetes.

Identifying costs of a novel service

The inputs to a service are far easier to cost than the outputs. A good service specification and implementation plan will enable all the costs associated with the service to be identified. These will include both fixed and variable costs. Fixed costs will be incurred regardless of the level of activity that the service delivers. These include all the set up costs such as recruitment, training and marketing as well as the costs of evaluation. There may be costs associated with assessment of competence to deliver the service, refurbishment costs and other capital expenditure for equipment. For example, a cardiovascular screening service which measures lipid and glucose levels will require a private room or area, plus testing equipment and may involve payment to a central quality assurance service.

Variable costs will depend on the level of activity of the service – how many people use it. These include the fee payable by the commissioner per intervention or patient and any tests, medicine or products provided, plus consumables. For example, a cardiovascular screening service which measures lipid and glucose levels will require consumables such as lancets, capillary blood tubes, testing strips and disposable gloves.

The balance between fixed and variable costs will depend on the individual service and if provided externally to the commissioning organisation, on how the payment structure is set up. The payments to providers commissioned to provide a service may be unit based or 'fee for item of service'. In this situation, the same fee may be paid for every patient/client who receives the service. An example is the Medicines Use Review service provided by community pharmacists in England and Wales. An alternative payment method is based on the number of patients/clients registered to receive the service, known as a per capita basis. There may also be the option to pay providers a fixed honorarium. Perhaps more difficult to establish, but arguably more relevant, is payment based on successful outcomes. For example, a smoking cessation service could offer a small fee to pharmacies for all clients who register, but a much larger fee for each client who is still not smoking at 12 weeks after initial registration. Many services could involve a mixture of these payment methods, with a fixed upfront honorarium type payment to cover fixed costs plus unit costs to reward activity.

In estimating the costs of a service the most valid information must be used, including using the local context rather than applying costs from external sources. For example, in estimating costs of accommodation for a training session, it makes sense to get the actual costs that will be incurred by contacting the venue rather than simply making a prediction. However, for some costs, it will be necessary to either obtain access to local health costs or derive costs from external sources. A good source for UK health and social costings is the publication *Unit Costs of Health and Social Care* produced from a DoH-funded programme based at the Personal Social Services Research Unit.[3]

Identifying potential cost savings from a novel service
Locally the public health unit and, in particular, the public health intelligence unit may be able to provide local costs for activities and treatments. These may be useful in estimating the cost benefits of services that prevent

NHS-related activity being needed, for example, GP appointments or admissions to hospital. However, it is worth noting that if a service prevents an acute admission, the full cost of avoiding that admission will never be recouped by the service due to the level of fixed costs associated with acute services and the fact that there will always be another person who will be admitted instead. Therefore there is a need to be realistic about the costs saved. That is not to say that avoiding an admission is not valued by the health service, it is simply that this value is not assessed in purely cost terms but more likely natural service outputs such as acute admissions avoided, percentage contribution to achieving health service targets. The service specification and implementation plan should help to identify all costs. Points to consider are listed in Box 9.6.

Box 9.6 *Points to consider in drafting a business case for a service*

- What are the capital costs of implementing and running the service, e.g. new buildings, development of consultation areas, new equipment?
- What are the staff costs of running the service, e.g. salaries, backfill for staff reallocated etc?
- Are there any training costs associated? (Remember to include the course fees, travel, accommodation and wages.)
- Are there any ongoing costs, e.g. registration fees, continuing professional development requirements, revalidation, equipment servicing and replacement?
- What are the costs associated with the intervention, e.g. medication, tests?
- What are the administration costs associated with the service?
- Can any costs be written off against savings? (Be careful as some apparent savings such as bed days saved in hospital are only theoretical, as the bed will be taken up by someone else; so although activity elsewhere in the healthcare system will increase, the bed will not remain empty.)

Governance of pharmacy services

Since the drive for increased efficiency in the NHS in the 1980s, there has been much discussion about how much is spent on healthcare and how to fund increasing expectation and demands from the health service. This focus on how much is spent on healthcare and the health gain derived from it is mirrored across the world.

As financial input to healthcare increases, questions are rightly asked about the outputs that will be generated. These are generally the tangible measurable health outputs that are the core function of the NHS. For example, how long does it take to get a hip replacement; if drug X is available in one health board area why isn't available in another?; what are the outcomes of coronary bypass operations at hospital X compared with Y?

Against this background, increasing emphasis has been placed on governance at the corporate level. This is how a healthcare organisation is directed and controlled, at its most senior levels, to achieve its objectives and meet the necessary standards of accountability, probity and openness. The concept of corporate governance was first defined by the London Stock Exchange Committee on Corporate Governance in the Cadbury Committee Report of 1992.[4] Corporate governance structures specify the distribution of rights and responsibilities within an organisation and define the framework of rules and procedures within which decision making takes place. Key aspects of corporate governance are:

- setting and achieving objectives
- being explicit about roles and responsibilities
- an emphasis on systems and process working
- upholding public service values
- managing clinical and financial risk
- including value for money in decision making.

For any service, both the provider and commissioner should be able to identify:

- how the service's aims and objectives contribute and map to the local healthcare organisation objectives
- how clinical responsibilities within the service are distributed and how legal liability for service delivery and outcomes are outlined
- clear explicit processes, often in the form of standard operating procedures or sets of standards, which describe the main pathways of service delivery
- where clinical and financial risks might occur and describe the nature of these.

Clinical governance as a term was first introduced to the NHS in 1998 with the publication of *A First Class Service: Quality in the NHS* in England[5] and *Designed to Care* in Scotland.[6] Clinical governance is defined as 'a framework through which NHS organisations are accountable for continuously improving the quality of their services and safeguarding high standards of care, by creating environments in which excellence in clinical care will flourish'.[5] The purpose and scope of clinical governance within the NHS was clearly described in guidance issued in 1998,[7] which stated that clinical governance will provide assurance to patients and practitioners that:

- quality of clinical care will drive decision making about the provision, organisation and management of services
- the planning and delivery of services will take full account of the perspectives of patients
- care delivered meets relevant standards
- unacceptable clinical practice will be detected and addressed.

The RPSGB describes a series of processes that make up clinical governance activity[8]:

- accountability
- audit
- clinical effectiveness
- continuing professional development
- patient and public involvement
- remedying underperformance
- risk management
- staff management.

Key to delivering clinical governance within service development are: clarity about the standards the service is trying to deliver, factors and processes that will enable this delivery, identification and mitigation of the risks associated with delivery, evaluation of the service to demonstrate that objectives have been met and procedures to identify and remedy sub-standard performance. Most of these have already been covered, but evaluation and audit of the service are further essential components.[2]

Service evaluation and audit

Evaluating a service

It may seem a little early to be considering evaluating a service before it is established, but evaluation is an essential part of service development, which can be overlooked. Evaluation should cover the range of service objectives including health improvement outcomes, process performance and client and provider satisfaction. It requires both time and resources and should be carefully planned. It is important to ensure a balance between evaluation and the delivery of the service. Defining how the service will be evaluated at the service development stage helps focus evaluation activity on the important aspects of outcome attainment and areas of risk in terms of service quality.

Evaluation may differ from many of the studies identified in the literature as providing evidence for developing the service in that the latter are determining whether a service can show a benefit and therefore constitute research. A literature search may also identify previous service evaluations, but it is important to understand that evaluation is more about whether a service works in practice. Once a service is well established, it may be appropriate to audit the quality of the service. The differences between research, evaluation and audit are shown in Table 9.1.

Table 9.1 Differentiating research, evaluation and audit[10]		
Research	**Clinical audit**	**Service evaluation**
The attempt to derive generalisable new knowledge including studies that aim to generate hypotheses as well as studies that aim to test them	Designed and conducted to produce information to inform delivery of best care	Designed and conducted solely to define or judge current care
Quantitative research – designed to test a hypothesis. Qualitative research – identifies/explores themes following established methodology	Designed to answer the question: 'Does this service reach a predetermined standard?'	Designed to answer the question: 'What standard does this service achieve?'
Addresses clearly defined questions, aims and objectives	Measures against a standard	Measures current service without reference to a standard
Quantitative research – may involve evaluating or comparing interventions, particularly new ones. Qualitative research – usually involves studying how interventions and relationships are experienced	Involves an intervention in use *only*. (The choice of treatment is that of the clinician and patient according to guidance, professional standards and/or patient preference.)	Involves an intervention in use *only*. (The choice of treatment is that of the clinician and patient according to guidance, professional standards and/or patient preference.)
Usually involves collecting data that are additional to those for routine care but may include data collected routinely. May involve treatments, samples or investigations additional to routine care	Usually involves analysis of existing data but may include administration of simple interview or questionnaire	Usually involves analysis of existing data but may include administration of simple interview or questionnaire
Quantitative research – study design may involve allocating patients to intervention groups	No allocation to intervention groups: the healthcare professional and patient have chosen intervention	No allocation to intervention groups: the healthcare professional and patient have chosen intervention
May involve randomisation	No randomisation	No randomisation
Reproduced with permission.		

A variety of methods can be used to evaluate services, including both qualitative and quantitative methods. It should be possible to determine whether the health-related outcomes outlined in the service specification have been achieved, but it is also important to obtain the views of service users, providers and others affected by the service on important aspects of how it is working. Although a research study in the area may have shown a service to have benefits, when implemented in a different locality by different people, in real-life situations, the effectiveness may be reduced. An evaluation should identify how effective a service is in reaching the target population. It is often very useful to obtain the views of people who are expected to use the service, rather than simply asking those who have already done so. This can often throw up potential barriers to access or expansion. An example of a service evaluation is given in Box 9.7.

Box 9.7 *An evaluation of a cardiovascular screening service in primary care*

Sefton Primary Care Trust has extremes of deprivation, with some areas being among the most deprived in England. The trust sought to commission a cardiovascular screening service from community pharmacists in deprived areas, developed the service specification, and provided training and all necessary equipment. An independent evaluation was commissioned separately. This evaluation incorporated the following.

1 In-depth telephone interviews with all service providers (community pharmacists) immediately prior to service delivery commencing, to determine:
   • views on the training provided
   • any further training undertaken or required
   • readiness to commence service delivery/further support required from the trust.
2 Questionnaires issued by pharmacists to service users, to determine:
   • how they learned about it
   • how they were invited for screening
   • suitability of venue
   • acceptability of information provided
   • perceived benefits
   • lifestyle changes made.
3 Telephone interviews with GPs to whom patients had been referred, to determine:
   • acceptability of the service
   • appropriateness of referrals.

4 Street surveys with potential service users, to determine:
  - awareness of the service and views on potential publicity
  - how they would wish to be invited for screening
  - suitability of venue
  - perceived benefits.
5 In-depth interviews with providers several months into service provision, to determine:
  - estimated time taken to perform screening, manage the data and issues arising
  - views on any changes required to the service specification, delivery methods and publicity
  - any additional costs associated with provision of the service.
6 Proportion of those screened with raised blood pressure, cholesterol and/or glucose and the frequency of high or moderate overall cardiovascular disease risk.
7 Proportion of people referred who attend for medical assessment and consequent treatments offered.

Once a service is established, with clear service standards in place, evaluation can then continue using audit, to assess how well the service is performing.

Auditing a service

Audit has been defined as 'a quality improvement process that seeks to improve patient care and outcomes through systematic review of care against explicit criteria and the implementation of change.'[9] Audit of a service should be a cyclical process (Figure 9.1) involving several stages.[9]

- *Step 1: Set criteria and agree standards.* It is important to set standards against which performance can be measured. These may come from external sources such as clinical guidelines or directly from the service specification. From these, indicators can be derived to measure how well the service matches those standards. Indicators are normally expressed as a percentage or a proportion of activity that meets the standard, e.g. a standard for a quit smoking programme might say that all smokers enrolled should have a record of their breath carbon monoxide taken three months after enrolling. For this standard an indicator could be defined as the percentage of smokers on the quit smoking programme who had a carbon monoxide measurement recorded three months after enrolment.

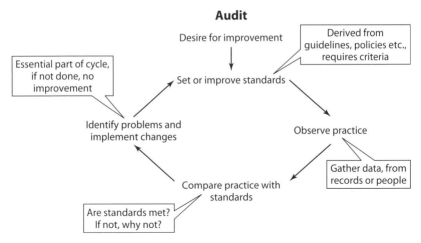

Figure 9.1 The audit cycle.

- *Step 2: Collect data.* Consideration needs to be given to the sampling frame, sample size, source of the data, issues of validity (accuracy) and reliability (consistency), data collection tools etc. This stage of an audit is essentially a survey of practice and should be planned as rigorously as a research project.
- *Step 3: Compare findings with standards.*
- *Step 4: Identify causes of non-achievement.* This is arguably the most important phase of an audit. If reasons for not achieving the standards are not identified then it will be difficult to implement change and improve care, the prime aim of clinical audit. In an audit of prescribing guidelines, consideration should be given to patients experiencing adverse effects necessitating withdrawal of therapy, contraindications, lack of awareness of the guidelines by practitioners etc.
- *Step 5: Implementing change.* If standards are not achieved, plans should be developed for altering practice. This is then followed by:
- *Step 6: Re-audit.*

References

1. National Primary and Care Trust Development Programme (2004). *The Commissioning Friend for PCTs: Whole system commissioning of acute services. National Primary and Care Trust Development Programme.* http://www.natpact.nhs.uk/uploads/CommissioningFriendMar04.pdf (accessed 9 December 2009).
2. McDonnell A, Wilson R, Goodacre S. Evaluating and implementing new services. *BMJ* 2006; 332: 109–112.
3. Curtis L. *Unit Costs of Health and Social Care.* Personal Social Services Research Unit, University of Kent, Canterbury, 2008. http://www.pssru.ac.uk/uc/uc2008contents.htm (accessed 9 December 2009).

4. Cadbury A (Chair). *Report of the Committee on the Financial Aspects of Corporate Governance*. London: The Committee on the Financial Aspects of Corporate Governance and Gee and Co., 1992.

5. Secretary of State for Health. *A First Class Service: Quality in the new NHS. 5*. Leeds: NHS Executive, 1998.

6. The Scottish Office. *Designed to Care: Renewing the National Health Service in Scotland*. Edinburgh: Scottish Executive, 1997.

7. Scottish Executive Health Department. *Guidance on Clinical Governance. NHS MEL* (1998) 75, 27 November 1998. Edinburgh: Scottish Executive.

8. Royal Pharmaceutical Society of Great Britain. *Clinical Governance* (homepage). London: RPSGB, 2009. http://www.rpsgb.org.uk/registrationandsupport/clinicalgovernance/ (accessed 9 December 2009).

9. Department of Health. *Clinical Governance* (homepage). London: Department of Health, 2009. http://www.dh.gov.uk/en/Publichealth/Patientsafety/Clinicalgovernance/index.htm (accessed 9 December 2009).

10. National Patient Safety Agency and National Research Ethics Service. *Defining Research*. London: NPSA/NRES, 2009. http://www.nres.npsa.nhs.uk/applications/apply/is-your-project-research/?locale=en (accessed 31 January 2010).

10

Risks and benefits

Peter Knapp, Janet Krska and Charles Morecroft

Most activities we undertake have both benefits and risks. We all face risk in our everyday lives, from running the risk of an accident through crossing the road to risks associated with sporting activities, from natural disasters or from taking medicines. Some activities carry greater risks than others, but risk taking behaviour is common, especially among young males, and is regarded as part of human nature. There may be a genetic predisposition towards risk taking, but it is also affected by the environment and other peoples' behaviour, such as one's peer group. Some evidence suggests that risk taking may be higher in more socioeconomically deprived groups, which may be related to greater peer pressure within these groups.

Similarly many interventions advocated by health professionals which aim to benefit individuals and improve public health are also associated with risk. Medicines are a common cause of risk, because of the huge variety of medicinal products and their potential for toxicity, combined with the fact that humans are involved in the various processes associated with using medicines. Being admitted to hospital can also have its associated risks. This is due to the major developments in technologies including medicines, increasing complexity of clinical processes and greater throughput of patients. There is the risk of hospital-acquired infection, the risks associated with procedures and treatments, not to mention the risk of errors.

A report published in 2000, *An Organisation with a Memory*, identified that errors were a common occurrence in the NHS, but that there was little evidence that staff learnt from these, to change working practices and prevent their recurrence.[1] This led directly to the establishment of the National Patient Safety Agency (NPSA), with a remit to collect, collate and review reports of incidents occurring within NHS premises or due to NHS services. A National Learning and Reporting Scheme (NLRS) has been established, which accepts reports from any NHS staff about patient safety incidents.[2] A patient safety incident is defined as: 'any unintended or unexpected incident that could have or did lead to harm.' These therefore include both errors and near misses. The reports are analysed to identify hazards and risks and to consider ways in which safety can be improved. The NPSA then recommends solutions, to ensure that lessons learnt from adverse events in one locality are proactively responded to by others within the NHS.

As part of clinical governance, pharmacists are required to regularly assess the risks associated with their practice and minimise risks to the public as part of the code of ethics. Communicating risk, along with communicating the potential benefits of changing behaviour or accepting interventions is an essential element of public health practice. Therefore this chapter covers how risks are perceived, how to communicate risks and benefits and how to assess and manage risks.

Risk perception

Risk can be explained as an unwanted outcome or the chances of that outcome occurring. Logic suggests that if the risk of a particular outcome is perceived to be highly associated with an activity, then it makes sense not to undertake the activity. The relationship between risk perception and behaviour is, however, not well understood and it does not follow that understanding of risk leads to a reduction in risky behaviour. For example, a survey in 1998 showed that junior house officers indulged in excess alcohol use, smoking and illicit drug use, despite a good awareness of the risks associated with these.[3] A study of students' behaviour showed that knowledge of the risks associated with a range of behaviours was not related to actual risk taking behaviour.[4] An understanding of how risks are perceived by patients and the public is important to ensure that both are communicated effectively.

Health professionals often believe they have a logical perspective of the risks and benefits of certain behaviours or of particular medicines, but may fail to appreciate that this perspective is not shared by patients or the public. For an individual, whether or not to undertake a potentially risky behaviour, including accepting a medical intervention, such as using a medicine, involves making a decision based on the chances of the unwanted outcome occurring and also to what extent that outcome would be detrimental to him/her. Risk has been described as having five dimensions (Table 10.1),[5] all of which are relevant to discussions about both lifestyle and medical interventions. It is suggested that the fifth dimension, value or perceived 'badness', is the most important and will have the greatest influence on an individual's decision as to whether or not to undertake or change a particular behaviour.

People generally underestimate or play down risks associated with lifestyle behaviours such as smoking or drinking alcohol, partly because they have chosen to undertake these – they are voluntary activities. Most people also perceive that the risk involved in playing dangerous sports, for example, is less

Table 10.1 Dimensions of risk in relation to potential adverse reactions (ADRs) from medicines

Dimension	Challenges	Examples in relation to ADRs
Identity	Not all potential outcomes (ADRs) may be known	Often the case for ADRs in newly marketed drugs, with limited use
Permanence	How long will the outcome last?	Will the ADR go away if the drug is stopped, or continued (tolerance)?
		Is the ADR likely to be permanent?
Timing	When will it occur?	Is it likely to occur on the first dose?
		Does it take a long time to develop?
		Could it occur on withdrawal of the drug?
Probability	How likely is an individual to experience the unwanted outcome?	Is it more or less likely if the drug is used regularly or long term?
		How do other medicines, other diseases, non-modifiable characteristics influence the probability?
Value	How important is it to the individual patient?	What is the patient's view of how bothersome the ADR is or may be?
		How will it affect their quality of life?

Adapted from reference 5.

than the average for the activity – 'it won't happen to me'. People who take risks through committing crime, through finance or in sport may perceive the risks associated with these as low, or that the risk is worth taking for the potential gain. Conversely risks associated with external activities, those imposed or suggested by others including health interventions or involuntary risks, such as food safety, may be perceived as high. Perception of risk is influenced by what health professionals may consider to be irrational beliefs. These may lead to behaviours which may also be regarded as irrational. Perceptions are developed over many years, informed by personal experiences and those of family and friends, social networks, behavioural norms and the media also plays an important role. All these perceptions of risk may influence subsequent behaviour. Individuals may also decide to undertake health-related behaviours because they don't wish to miss an opportunity (such as the chance of screening), have trust in technology or in a health professional, fear the consequences of not undertaking the behaviour or feel that it is their right to receive a particular intervention. Different models have been developed to describe health-related behaviour, the most well-known of

Table 10.2 Factors that influence risk acceptance

Factor increasing acceptance	Example	Factor decreasing acceptance	Example
Voluntary	Choosing to use mobile phone while driving	Involuntary	Inability to influence siting of nuclear power plant
Control	Choosing to eat unhealthy foods	No control	Lack of information about food sources
Natural	Choosing to live in area at risk of natural disaster	Technological	Choosing to live near chemical plant
High probability, low consequences	Heartburn with an NSAID	Low probability, high consequences	Stevens-Johnson syndrome with an NSAID
Familiar	Well-established drug	Non-familiar	Newly marketed drug
Involves adults	Taking prophylactic antimalarials for holiday	Involves children	Vaccinating with MMR

Adapted from reference 6.
NSAID = non-steroidal anti-inflammatory drug; MMR = measles, mumps, rubella vaccine.

which is probably the Health Belief Model (see Chapter 11). This includes perceived susceptibility to disease as a factor influencing the likelihood of taking action to change behaviour. Some key factors that affect the acceptance of risk are shown in Table 10.2.

Patients and the public may have difficulties in understanding risks described to them by health professionals, even if described using methods advocated as best practice. They may estimate their own risk based on the risks associated with something similar, perhaps a previous intervention. If there has been a lot of publicity about a particular risk, it may be over-estimated. Conversely underestimation may occur if individuals perceive themselves to be knowledgeable or even invulnerable. Small risks may also be underestimated, while large risks may be overestimated. These influences are described in greater detail in relation to medicines use in this chapter.

Risks and benefits associated with medicines

Patients need to be informed about both risks and benefits of medicines, for three reasons:

- They need to make informed decisions about medicines.
- They have a right to understandable information about the potential harms of medicines.

- Only if the patient is able to identify a side effect early and act upon it, can the impact of side effects be reduced.

The most likely source of information is the package leaflet now required by European law to accompany every licensed medicine.[7] The European Union (EU) proposed that the chance of side effects should be indicated by the use of verbal terms, such as 'rare' and 'common'. As described later, research shows that these terms produce gross misunderstanding by patients, which has led to a focus on the best method of describing the likelihood of side effects. Tools and aids are available to support professionals in informing people about the risks and benefits of treatments.[8] However, many people are not equipped to understand, retain and use risk information, which can be complex and threatening.[9]

Most patients want to know about side effects and the chance of them occurring. Berry et al.[10] asked participants what they would want to know about an antibiotic being prescribed for them using 16 categories of information. They found that information about side effects was the most sought after category (followed by knowing what the medicine does, any lifestyle changes that they would need to make and how it should be taken). However, doctors' ratings (when prescribing the antibiotic) were quite different: information about side effects and what the medicine actually does were both given low rankings.

Influences on perceptions of risks and benefits

An individual patient's understanding of information about the risks and benefits of treatment with a medicine (and their subsequent decision about the treatment) are both influenced by other factors. These may include their prior beliefs about the medicine, their emotions and the values they place on both the positive and negative outcomes of taking the medicine. In one study participants were asked to imagine being prescribed either penicillin (for a chest infection) or ibuprofen (for a bad back). They were then asked to estimate the chance of getting any side effect, and each of two named side effects for the medicine.[11] The results revealed an overestimation of the chance of getting any side effect (26% for penicillin compared with a reported incident rate of 18%) and a larger overestimation of the chance of the individual side effects. For example, renal damage was estimated at 15% in people taking ibuprofen compared with the reported incident rate of less than 0.1%. What is equally striking is the large variation in participants' estimates.

Information that practitioners provide to patients may conflict with pre-existing beliefs. This links to the 'Beliefs about Medicines Scale', which was developed to measure people's estimates of the harmful effects of medicines both generally and about specific medicines.[12] The scale has been applied to many clinical areas and again the variation among participants is striking.

Increasing access to web-based information and changes in the media reporting of health mean that patients are likely to read or hear more than a single account of the medicines they are taking. As a result, the information provided by professionals is likely to be only one of several sources of information patients can access, perhaps requiring them to reconcile apparently conflicting pieces of information, including their own experiences of taking medicines. They may not always make the decision desired by professionals or, to put it differently, the one that professionals themselves would have made. However, the values held by patients are powerful and may swamp statistical considerations of risk and benefit. For example, patients with rheumatoid arthritis may be unwilling to accept the chance of medicines' toxic effects, although the medicines might be highly beneficial.[13] Young people are much more concerned about getting acne as a side effect compared with doctors who consider this side effect to be minor.[10]

Information about risks and benefits may be presented to the patient in a rational way but it may be hard for them to make a decision entirely without emotion. Lowenstein[14] argues that, when the patient's emotions and rational thoughts are conflicted, the emotions will be dominant. This will be particularly important when patients are making decisions about treatments in highly emotive illnesses, such as those that are life threatening.

Communicating risks and benefits

In discussing risks with patients, it is important not to forget that there may also be risks associated with not undertaking the activity. So while the risks associated with taking a medicine may involve the possibility of experiencing an adverse drug reaction, the risks of not taking the medicine may be pain, disability, disease or death. It is essential to explain options available to enable individuals to make their own decisions, while maintaining respect for their perspective and right to refuse treatment or change behaviour. The way the discussion is carried out can have an influence on the decision reached by the individual. The relationship between health professional and patient, although ideally based on openness, trust and good communication, may often be paternalistic – 'doctor knows best'. This derives from the fact that in general patients are less well informed about health interventions or the risks associated with behaviours, putting the health professional in the position of expert. Body language, terminology and tone of voice are all important ways in which the health professional may bias discussions in favour of their perceptions of risk. For example, a health professional may describe the risk of stomach upset with aspirin as 'minor', or the risk of muscle pain with a statin as 'justifiable, for the benefit to health'. However, this may in fact be their perception of risk, which could have undue influence on the patient who currently has no symptoms, trying to decide whether or not to accept the suggested intervention.

Methods of conveying risk and benefit

There are many different options to choose from when conveying information about risk and benefit to patients. However, there are four main approaches: the use of words, or numbers, or graphs, or some combination of these. Examples of each of the four approaches are given below. The approaches vary in the extent to which they have been evaluated – some recommendations have had little formal evaluation. Furthermore, some of the examples that have been evaluated, have proved not to be very effective.

Using words

The EU's recommended scale of verbal terms for risk ranges from 'very common' (for rates of more than 1 in 10) to 'very rare' (for rates of less than 1 in 10 000). The use of these verbal terms can lead to a large overestimation of risk when compared with the equivalent numerical expressions.[15] For example, patients taking a statin interpreted the term 'common', when used to describe the risk of the side effect constipation, to have a mean rate of occurrence of 34%, much higher than its actual incidence. The use of the terms was also linked to increased estimates of the medicine's severity and, importantly, a reduction in the number of participants who said they would take the medicine.

Other verbal scales pre-date the EU recommendation, including that proposed by Calman.[16] It uses seven points ranging from high (more than 1 in 100) to negligible (less than 1 in 1 million). Again this scale led to significant overestimation of risk, particularly in the lower frequency bands (which are likely to be used mostly for more harmful side effects).[17] Evaluations of the EU and Calman scales also show considerable variation among participants (Table 10.3). This means it is hard to achieve a common understanding of what numerical values (or range of values) are attached to frequency terms.

Table 10.3 Verbal terms to describe risk		
EC guideline descriptor	Mean (SD) estimate from study participants (%)	Frequency assigned by EU (%)
Very common	65 (24.3)	>10
Common	45 (22.2)	1–10
Uncommon	18 (13.0)	0.1–1
Rare	8 (7.5)	0.01–0.1
Very rare	4 (6.7)	<0.01

Using numbers

If words don't work well, then a simple option is to use numbers and here there are several alternatives. Using percentages is one option, so that the chance of benefit or risk of side effect might be given as 5%, for example. However, percentages are not understood by a significant minority of people. In a much-cited study, Gigerenzer asked people to explain the meaning of '40%'.[18] Although around three-quarters of respondents could explain the term correctly, the remainder were inaccurate, with common responses being 'one in four' or 'one in forty'. Other studies looking at ways of expressing side effect risk also suggest some difficulty in interpreting, and a reluctance to use, percentages of less than 1%.[19] This will cause problems for conveying medicine side effect risks, given that many have a low incidence rate.

Gigerenzer advocates the use of 'natural frequencies', that is whole numbers related to individuals receiving a treatment. He has shown that presenting natural frequencies, e.g. 'Out of 100 people taking this medicine, 1 will get side effect X' is more likely to be understood than the percentage equivalent.[18] It is thought that the natural frequency expression is easier to interpret because it is concrete, since it relates to a defined group of persons out of which one person is affected by a stated outcome. By comparison, percentages are abstract and lack a 'reference class'.

When two or more risks are to be presented, possibly to communicate treatment options, research suggests that people find the risks easier to understand when a common denominator is used. For example, 20 out of 1000 and 5 out of 1000 are more likely to be understood than 1 in 50 and 1 in 200.[20,21]

The Medicines and Healthcare products Regulatory Agency in the UK advocates the use of a combined words and frequencies approach, e.g. 'common' (affects more than 1 in 100 persons)'.[22] This combined expression needs evaluation with one study to date suggesting that the verbal terms in a combined expression may dominate other included information, i.e. the numbers.[23] Another numerical option is to use the *number needed to treat* (NNT, for benefits) or *number needed to harm* (NNH, for harms/side effects) expression (see Chapter 7). These expressions depend on there being a comparison – either between two treatments, or between a treatment and no treatment (or placebo). This format has been used increasingly in recent years[24] and one study suggests that it is better understood by patients than other forms of risk expression.[25] The need for NNT or NNH expressions to draw on two treatment arms means that this approach becomes unwieldy and is much less useful when having to describe several frequencies. Further research is needed to determine whether the population understand NNH and NNT and if they find them acceptable.

Using graphs

Graphs provide another option. However, there has been little evaluation of their use in displaying data on medicine risks. Graphs have been used more extensively in decision aids to show the benefits of two (or more) treatment options. One widely used method involves the use of 'icon arrays', also known as a 'Paling palette'. This is a grid of 100 (or 1000) faces (or stick figures) to convey information on the chances of positive and negative outcomes.[21] However, recent work showed that faces grids were less easy for people to interpret than a coloured bar chart,[26] a tendency that is also reported in a systematic review of work in this area.[27] This review identifies that common approaches to displaying risk graphically include bar charts and pie charts, with linear graphs being used, in particular, to show two or more incidence rates on one scale. The limitation of using graphs of any type is space on the page: too small and their impact will be negligible. They may also depend on colour for interpretation and impact, an important concern given that production costs will restrict much patient information to black and white printing. Finally, graphs conveying numerical data ought to be used to give an overall impression or a simple message; they are generally less useful when conveying lots of detail.

Key factors in communicating risk and benefit

There are a number of key effects which must be borne in mind when communicating information about risk and benefit. These include relative and absolute data, framing, context and heuristics (mental short cuts).

Heuristics

People often use heuristics when making judgements. The use of heuristics when making judgements about probability can lead to the correct answer but is associated with systematic errors or biases. One such example is the availability heuristic, used by people when asked to judge the frequency of an event. People using the availability heuristic make an estimate based on how easy or difficult it is to recall particular instances. As a result, such judgements can be influenced by how readily instances can be recalled. One study showed that causes of death that attract more publicity (such as murder) are judged more frequent than those that attract less publicity (e.g. suicide, some types of cancer), but which are in fact much more frequent.[28]

Relative versus absolute risk

People's judgements of risk and benefit information are also influenced by its presentation. One example is whether absolute or relative forms are used. The relative risk reduction (RRR) compares the risk for one group with that for another group (see Chapter 7). By contrast the absolute risk reduction (ARR) indicates a difference between two risk frequencies. For example, a risk reduction from 6% to 3% can be expressed as 'reduced by 50%' (RRR) or as a 'reduction of 3%' (ARR). A review of more than 200 media reports for three medicines found that a large majority (83%) presented benefits only as RRR, with 15% using both relative and absolute benefits and 2% communicating only absolute benefits.[29]

The use of the relative form of risk increase in the media has been attributed as the cause of the 1995 contraceptive 'pill scare'. New data at the time showed that women taking the third generation contraceptive pill were about twice as likely to be affected by thromboembolism. This (relative form) was reported in national newspapers without reference to the absolute data, which showed that the risks, although doubled, remained very low. In fact the risk of thromboembolism was increased from about 15 cases per 100 000 pill users to 25 cases.[30] Publicity led to many women stopping taking the pill, resulting in an increase in unwanted pregnancies and terminations. Ironically, the risk of thromboembolism in pregnancy is four to five times higher than in women taking the pill.

It is not only patients who are influenced by relative risk forms: one study found that physicians are more likely to prescribe medical treatments if risk reductions are communicated in relative formats.[31]

Context and framing

People's interpretations of risk information are also influenced by the context in which the judgement is made. One study reviewed 450 informed consent decisions and found that judgements of probability (expressed verbally) were influenced by the severity of the consequences.[32] In the context of medicine side effects, people's interpretation of verbal terms, such as 'common', depend on the severity of the side effect being described,[33] and whether the medicine is being prescribed for an adult or a one-year-old child.[34]

Judgements are also influenced by whether the information is framed positively or negatively. For example, presenting patients with a video describing the risks of angioplasty using positive framing (i.e. as 99% safe) resulted in more opting for the treatment than when it was framed negatively (i.e. the chance of complication being 1%).[35] Doctors have also been shown to be affected by information framing: when information was framed in terms of risk of dying it significantly reduced the likelihood that doctors would recommend radiation therapy over surgery.[36]

Similar effects have been found in relation to loss and gain framing. Framing information in terms of losses tends to be more influential than framing the same information in terms of gains. Thus, when explaining to people about some form of health screening, telling them about the risks of not being screened (*loss framing*) leads to a greater uptake of screening than telling them about the benefits from being screened (*gain framing*).[37]

Communicating uncertainty

A significant issue in communicating risks and benefits is the confidence you have in the data that are used to generate the risk and benefit estimates. The method of data generation is important: was it a prospective study, or post-marketing surveillance? How many participants were included in the study? These issues will impact on confidence, both in a formal sense in terms of the width of the statistical confidence intervals, and less formally in terms of the credibility of the study and its data.

Post-marketing surveillance data can indicate the type of side effects a medicine causes but establishing a rate is almost impossible because there is so much uncertainty about the number of people taking the medicine. However, this uncertainty may be difficult to communicate to patients. Lack of certainty or knowledge is not something people necessarily understand or accept.

Data from randomised controlled trials and meta-analysis within a systematic review are more useful, since the numbers of people taking the medicine are known, and so a rate (whether of harm or benefit) can be calculated. However, trials can be of limited use for adverse drug reactions: such events in a trial may be counted and reported but often not in detail. Perhaps of more concern, trials tend to have relatively short follow-up periods, thus reducing their validity as indicators of patient outcomes in general.

People's ability to understand uncertainty varies, whether the risks presented concern treatment harm or benefit (or both). There is a common pattern emerging from a number of studies, to show that people with low levels of numeracy skills are less able to estimate risks, or to accurately extract risk estimates from information presented to them.[38,39] The numeracy required to understand risks may be seen as an aspect of functional health literacy, which Nutbeam[40] defines as 'sufficient basic skills in reading and writing to be able to function effectively in everyday situations.' When patients' numeracy abilities vary, it is crucial that practitioners check to ensure that any risk information provided to patients has been understood.

However good the data source for risk and benefit estimates, one aspect of uncertainty is inevitable, that is, the uncertainty associated with translating data drawn from a population to individuals. The rates of harmful and beneficial effects of treatment are calculated by drawing on population data, meaning that the precise effects for an individual are inevitably uncertain. As for rate calculation, this lack of certainty may be difficult for some patients to accept. Large trials and studies with prospective longitudinal designs can indicate risk factors that will increase (or decrease) the chance of a particular outcome occurring in a particular patient. Furthermore, future developments in genetic profiling may increase the amount of information available, but a lack of absolute certainty will remain with most harms and benefits associated with treatments.

Medicines supply as a source of risk

In addition to adverse drug reactions, medicines account for 10% of all incidents reported to the NPSA through the NLRS, with over 70 000 incidents reported during 2008/09.[41] Adverse events caused by medicines occur in both secondary care and the community, and although community pharmacies are still a very minor source of reports to the NLRS, medicines are the largest cause of incidents reported through primary care.[37] The medicine supply process involves a number of stages: prescribing, dispensing, preparation, administration and monitoring. Pharmacists can be involved in all stages, but most frequently in prescribing, dispensing and preparation. Whether working in primary or secondary care, part of the pharmacist's role is to identify and address errors in prescribing and, of course, they may prescribe themselves. Prescribing errors occur at a rate of between 1.5 % and 9% in secondary care[42] and 7.5% in primary care.[43] However, pharmacists themselves are responsible for errors or near misses in dispensing, which have been found to occur at a rate of 26 per 100 000 prescriptions dispensed in community pharmacy.[44] Errors were most frequently caused by selection but were also associated with organisational factors, such as distractions, workload, staffing and skill mix. Such organisational factors are known as latent errors (see page 165).

Assessing risks associated with medicines supply

A risk assessment is simply an assessment of what could cause harm, together with identifying ways of reducing the risk. The Health and Safety Executive has identified five steps to safety within the workplace:

- Identify the risks.
- Decide who may be harmed and how.
- Evaluate the risks and decide on precautions.
- Record what has been found, precautions agreed and implement these.
- Review the assessment and update regularly or as needed.

In relation to medicines supply, many risks have been identified by the NPSA. These include products with similar names (generic or trade) or similar packaging, aimed primarily at maintaining a corporate brand image. The NPSA works with manufacturers towards reducing these problems, by recommending changes such as greater colour differences, larger fonts for product strengths or the addition of extra text on packaging. However, individual pharmacists also need to assess risks within their workplace and manage these risks.

Assessing risks usually involves making a judgement about their importance. This is most often done by first estimating the likelihood of a particular risk occurring, then considering the impact of that occurrence on patients or the organisation or both. The two are then multiplied to calculate the overall risk. To manage risks, the plans for preventing the occurrence are then added and a residual risk calculated, assuming the plan is implemented (see Table 10.4 for an example of how this works).

Injectable medicines are particularly risky, because of the large number of errors associated with their preparation and administration. The NPSA recommends that an annual risk assessment should be carried out by a pharmacist and a clinician for all clinical areas where injectable medicines are prepared and administered. This should examine the products themselves as well as how they are actually prepared and administered. A risk assessment tool is available to assist with this, which examines both product and procedural factors.[45] Product factors which may increase risk include: serious effect if given in wrong dose or by wrong route, product requires dilution, complex calculation or reconstitution required before use, need to use part of container or syringe driver. Assessment of the procedures involves looking for poor practices, so that these can be addressed. These include lack of instructions for correct preparation, using unlabelled filled syringes, preparing cytotoxic or total parenteral nutrition products outside the pharmacy and mixing drugs within one syringe.

Managing risks associated with medicines supply

Managing the risks associated with dispensing requires an understanding of why errors occur in the first place. There are two main theories of error: blame theory and systems theory.[46] The blame theory suggests that individuals are at fault, perhaps because of being particularly accident-prone, having insufficient training or practice, needing to improve their skills or knowledge. It may also apportion blame owing to forgetfulness, inattention, negligence or even recklessness. This approach does little to encourage reporting or learning from errors so is completely discouraged within the NHS. Conversely the systems approach recognises that human actions do inevitably sometimes result in errors and that the conditions and procedures within which they work may contribute to these errors. This approach is that adopted by the NPSA.

A four-stage model was developed by Reason,[46] which hypothesised that latent failure, failure by management/organisation, resulted in poor working conditions. These in turn could lead to active failures by those doing the actual tasks, such as dispensing, but there are defences against this, helping to prevent errors from occurring. Reason described four types of error:

- slips or attentional failures
- lapses or memory failures

Table 10.4 Example of using a risk assessment method to improve public health advice provision

Stage 1 Assessing current risk

Potential risk	Initial risk assessment			Mitigation	
	Probability	Impact	Overall	Plan with timescale	Responsibility
Opportunistic brief interventions not offered	4	3	12	Develop and deliver training within 3 months	Superintendent pharmacist
Free emergency hormonal contraception not routinely available	5	3	15	Check accreditation status of all locum pharmacists as soon as possible	Store manager
CVD screening not available	5	4	15	One pharmacist to undertake training and accreditation	Regular pharmacist

Stage 2 Assessing impact of risk management strategy

Desired outcome	Residual risk			Review
	Probability	Impact	Overall	Date (months)
Staff regularly offer brief interventions	2	2	4	6
All locums accredited before being employed	2	1	3	3
CVD screening available most days	3	2	6	6

Scoring scales

Probability		Impact		Overall risk	
1	Very unlikely	1	Insignificant	Score between 1 and 6	Green – no action required
2	Unlikely	2	Minor		
3	Possible	3	Moderate	Score between 8 and 12	Amber – action required
4	Probable	4	High		
5	Very likely	5	Unacceptable	Score between 16 and 25	Red – immediate action required

CVD = cardiovascular disease.

- mistakes, due to poor execution of a good process, or good execution of a poor process
- violations, or deliberate deviations from the process.

The last type can be due to individuals feeling that they do not need to conform to the procedures, the procedures do not apply in a particular instance or it becomes routine practice not to follow the procedures. Clearly there is a need to move away from the blame theory to ensure that incidents are routinely reported to enhance organisation learning. On the other hand, staff may be uncomfortable in exposing weakness in the system if this involves challenging the organisational hierarchy. Similarly, an 'open and fair' culture towards reporting as advocated by the NPSA is not so easy to encourage, since pharmacists can and have been prosecuted for a dispensing error.

Addressing latent failures may result in greater improvements in error rates than dealing only with active failures, since the former may result in conditions under which it is difficult to avoid active failures. This could include routinely being understaffed or ill-equipped or being asked to use poorly designed or unworkable procedures. The adoption of electronic prescribing has the potential to reduce prescribing errors, although research suggests that it does not eliminate them.[47] Pharmacists are required to have established standard operating procedures (SOPs) for dispensing, which should be designed to minimise the risk of error. These should be designed with the involvement of all staff involved in the dispensing process, so ensuring their practicality as well as likelihood of adoption. Automated dispensing systems have been installed in many UK hospital pharmacies and in some community pharmacies elsewhere, which have also been shown to reduce, but not eliminate, dispensing errors.

Of course a further important role of pharmacists is in the checking of prescriptions written by others. Although this topic is not within the scope of this book, one example of how risks can be minimised is in the field of oncology, where errors could have very serious consequences. The British Oncology Pharmacists' Association have produced standards for verifying the prescribing of systemic anticancer therapies, which outline the key checks that a pharmacist must undertake prior to preparation and supply of the product.[48]

Developing a safety culture

Reporting errors is a vital part of every health professional's job and the NPSA's national reporting and learning service encourages this. Research undertaken in 2005 showed that both pharmacists and support staff were, however, very unlikely to report incidents to the NPSA or even within the pharmacy.[44] A safety culture is required in health organisations, including pharmacies, but this is a relatively new concept. The NPSA advocates using the Manchester patient safety profile, which is a tool designed to enable organisations to assess their progress in developing such a culture.[49] This tool has been adapted for use in community pharmacies.[44]

Managing risk often involves changing procedures. This may be very simple or require extensive collaborative work. Simple solutions to reducing errors resulting from products with similar names or packaging could be placing them in different locations within the dispensary, or putting up warning signs indicating products should be double checked before dispensing. Reducing the risks associated with injectable medicines could include the simple provision of written procedures for preparing and administering medicines to be available in all clinical areas. However, it may involve the need to develop a new service or make radical changes to procedures within the pharmacy. Such major change itself requires to be managed adequately. Public health practitioners are frequently involved in managing changes to NHS services, whether for the purpose of reducing risk or other reasons.

Managing change

It has been said that the NHS changes all the time, but stays the same. Obviously interventions and practices have indeed changed over the years and there have been frequent structural or organisational changes, yet many behaviours and attitudes remain the same. A frequent problem within the NHS is the failure to learn from previous experiences of others, which stifles development because of the constant need to 're-invent the wheel'. Developing a safety culture is typical of the change that is required, as is moving from a 'national illness service' to a 'national wellness service' through delivering public health interventions, rather than responding to already established disease.

Increasingly it is recognised that it is important for staff to understand how to deal with continuous change and development. Implementing new services to maximise benefits to patients and minimise risks, as shown in Chapter 9, will inevitably involve changes to existing practices, but also an ability to measure the effectiveness of processes and services. One important way of avoiding 're-inventing the wheel' is to search the literature, but herein lies another problem in that not all development work is published or publicised. Subsequent chapters will highlight much of the evidence currently available on the effectiveness of public health services involving pharmacists. Even if effective new processes and services are identified from the literature, you still have to implement these in your own practice.

There are many different theories about how to implement changes to practice and also a body of evidence showing what works. A large amount of material on managing change within the NHS is available, covering many different methods, a few of which are briefly described here.

Seven S model

This model is a way of thinking holistically about resources and competences available within a team, to ensure they are helping achieve its goals. It could be used for example, in developing a novel service to screen patients for cardiovascular risk. The model includes seven interrelated aspects: staff, skills, structure, systems, strategy, style of management and shared beliefs.

- *Staff:* are the right staff in place in terms of numbers and different grades to allow the service to be developed? If not what do we need to do to change this?
- *Skills:* what are the key skills are required and do we have them? What training is needed and where can we obtain this?
- *Structure:* does the organisation's structure make the most of the staff and skills we have to facilitate this new service?
- *Systems:* are all the vital systems and procedures in place to enable this service to happen?
- *Strategy:* do we have a clear goal of what we hope to achieve with the new service?
- *Style of management:* what is the predominant management style and does it empower staff to support the service?
- *Shared beliefs:* do the staff fully support the service as being an important development within our pharmacy?

Five 'whys'

Trying to change your practice because you have identified problems such as a high dispensing error rate or a failure to deliver opportunistic health advice to customers first requires an analysis of why this happens. Undertaking a root cause analysis is the first step in this process. Five 'whys' is simple tool, which can help to identify the root cause of a problem. An example of how this works is given in Box 10.1. Root cause analysis often results in the shifting of blame for an error or failure from an individual to the organisation. This tool is particularly useful when similar errors or failures keep recurring.

Action research, using 'Plan, Do, Study, Act' cycles

Action research is a method of involving practitioners in developing solutions to problems within their organisation, through continuous development and

Box 10.1 *An example of using five 'whys' for analysing the root cause of a failure to deliver*

A large community pharmacy has recently established a smoking cessation service, including one-to-one and group sessions and staff are expected to promote this service to potential clients at every opportunity. The service involves an initial chat to the specialist pharmacist who will assess the client's readiness to change smoking habits, then record their name, if they are willing, for future contact. The specialist pharmacist notices that Jane, a medicines counter assistant (MCA), has just sold a cough mixture but did not ask about smoking or mention the service.

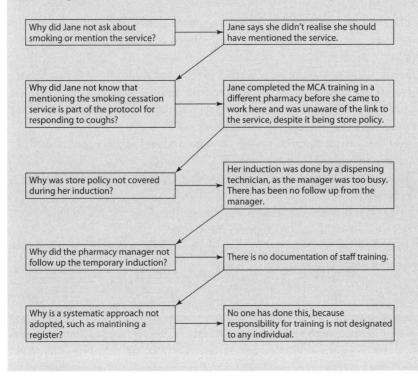

testing. It requires the involvement of individuals affected by or who may be contributing to a problem. The first stage is to gather information about the problem, then identify the causes, suggest ideas to improve things, test these out on a small scale, then gather more data to find out if the suggested solutions worked and act on the results. This may mean trying different changes or, if successful, going a little further with changes, perhaps involving

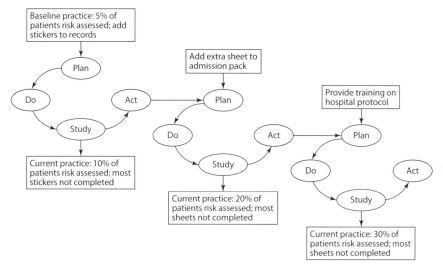

Figure 10.1 Using PDSA cycles to effect changes to risk assessment for venous thromboembolism. Assessing medical patients admitted to hospital for venous thromboembolism is now required. Guidance has been issued by the Department of Health and a hospital protocol developed. However, an audit shows that this is not taking place, which could result in death and disability from venous thromboembolism during hospital admission. The figure shows how it is necessary to implement a series of small actions, together with gathering data on how these have impacted on practice, before sufficient change is achieved.

more people or implementing them on a larger scale or for a longer period. These repeated cycles of development are known as 'plan, do, study, act' (PDSA) cycles (Figure 10.1).

Audit

Although perhaps more familiar to pharmacists as a means of determining whether clinical guidelines are being used, audit is in fact a method for improving practices and services which leads to an improvement. Audit requires a standard, against which practice is measured by gathering data, the implementation of changes to practice and subsequent re-audit. Repeated audit cycles are rarely used in practice, many audits simply consisting of the initial data gathering and comparison to standards. One aspect of audit which is most frequently omitted is finding out why standards are not being met. This aspect can be undertaken using five whys or other similar methods of root cause analysis and changes can be implemented using plan, do, study, act cycles. Importantly whatever changes are needed to improve practices and services, it is essential to involve all relevant staff, teams and agencies, hence applying the principles of working with others (see Chapter 8). An ability to influence others may be a key skill required to make changes happen. Influencing skills are covered in Chapter 14.

References

1. Department of Health. *An Organisation With a Memory: A report from an expert working group on learning from adverse events in the NHS*. London: Department of Health, 2000. http://www.dh.gov.uk/en/Publicationsandstatistics/Publications/PublicationsPolicyAndGuidance/DH_4065083

2. National Patient Safety Agency. National Reporting and Learning Service (homepage). http://www.nrls.npsa.nhs.uk/

3. Birch D, Ashton H, Kamali F. Alcohol, drinking, illicit drug use and stress in junior house officers in north-east England. *Lancet* 1998; 352: 785–786.

4. Cook PA, Bellis MA. Risk behaviour and health knowledge. *Public Health* 2001; 115: 54–61.

5. Bogardus ST, Holmboe E, Jekel JF. Perils, pitfalls and possibilities in talking about medical risk. *JAMA* 1999; 281: 1037–1041.

6. Risk and Regulation Advisory Council. *A Practical Guide to Risk Communication*. London: RRAC, 2009. http://www.berr.gov.uk/files/file51458.pdf

7. European Commission. *European Commission Council Directive 92/27/EEC* (OJ NoL 113 of 30.4.1992, p.8) m1992.

8. Cranney A. Decision aids in clinical practice. *BMJ* 2004; 329: 39–40.

9. Berry D. *Risk, Communication and Health Psychology*. Maidenhead: Open University Press, 2004.

10. Berry DC, Michas IC, Gillie T *et al*. What do patients want to know about their medicines and what do doctors want to tell them? A comparative study. *Psychol Health* 1997; 12: 467–480.

11. Knapp P, Coppack Z, Raynor DK. *What Do People Think Is the Likelihood of Harm and Benefit from Two Common Medicines?* Presented at the Health Services Research and Pharmacy Practice conference, London, 2004. http://www.hsrpp.org.uk/abstracts/2004_46.shtml

12. Horne R, Weinman J. Patients' beliefs about prescribed medicines and their role in adherence to treatment in chronic physical illness. *J Psychosomat Res* 1999; 47: 555–567.

13. Frankael L, Bogardus S, Concato J *et al*. Risk communication in rheumatoid arthritis. *J Rheumatol* 2003; 30: 443–448.

14. Lowenstein GF, Weber EU, Hsee CK *et al*. Risk as feelings. *Psychol Bull* 2001; 127: 267–286.

15. Knapp P, Raynor DK, Berry DC. Comparison of two methods of presenting risk information to patients about the side effects of medicines. *Qual Saf Health Care* 2004; 13: 176–180.

16. Calman KC. Cancer, science and society and the communication of risk. *BMJ* 1996; 313: 799–802.

17. Berry DC, Knapp P, Raynor DK. Provision of information about drug side effects to patients. *Lancet* 2002; 359: 853–854.

18. Gigerenzer G. *Reckoning With Risk*. London: Penguin, 2002.

19. Knapp P, Gardner PH, Carrigan N *et al*. Perceived risk of medicine side effects in users of a patient information website: a study of the use of verbal descriptors, percentages and absolute frequencies. *Br J Health Psychol* 2009; 14: 579–594.

20. Grimes DA, Snively GR. Patients' understanding of medical risks: implications for genetic counseling. *Obstet Gynecol* 1999; 93: 910–914.

21. Paling J. Strategies to help patients understand risks. *BMJ* 2003; 327: 745–748.

22. Medicines and Healthcare products Regulatory Agency. *Always Read the Leaflet: Getting the best information with every medicine. Report of the Committee on Safety of Medicines Working Group on Patient Information*. London: TSO, 2005.

23. Knapp P, Raynor DK, Woolf E *et al*. Communicating the risk of side effects to patients: an evaluation of UK regulatory recommendations. *Drug Saf* 2009; 32: 837–849.

24. Anon. Calculating and using NNTs. *Bandolier*, February 2003. http://www.medicine.ox.ac.uk/bandolier/Extraforbando/NNTextra.pdf (accessed 22 February 2010).

25. Misselbrook D, Armstrong D. Patients' responses to risk information about the benefits of treating hypertension. *Br J Gen Pract* 2001; 51: 276–279.

26. Knapp P, Wanklyn P, Raynor DK *et al.* Developing and testing a patient information booklet for thrombolysis used in acute stroke. *Int J Pharm Pract* epub ahead of print, doi: 10.1111/ j.2042-7174. 2010.00060.

27. Ancker J, Senathirajah Y, Kukafka R *et al.* Design features of graphs in health risk communication: a systematic review. *J Am Med Inf Assoc* 2006; 13: 608–618.

28. Lichtenstein S, Slovic P, Fischoff B *et al.* Judged frequency of lethal events. *J Exp Psychol* 1978; 4: 551–578.

29. Moynihan R, Bero L, Ross-Degnon D *et al.* Coverage by the news media of the benefits and risks of medication. *N Engl J Med* 2000; 342: 1645–1650.

30. Berry DC, Raynor DK, Knapp P *et al.* Official warnings on thromboembolism risk with oral contraceptives fail to inform users adequately. *Contraception* 2002; 66: 305–307.

31. Lacy C, Barone J, Suh D *et al.* Impact of presentation of research results on likelihood of prescribing medications in patients with left ventricular presentations. *Am J Cardiol* 2001; 87: 203–207.

32. Merz JF, Druzdel MJ, Mazur DJ. Verbal expressions of probability in informed consent litigation. *J Med Decis Making* 1991; 1: 273–281.

33. Berry DC, Raynor DK, Knapp P. Communicating risk of medication side effects: an empirical evaluation of EU recommended terminology. *Psychol Health Med* 2003; 8: 251–263.

34. Berry DC. Interpreting information about medication side effects: differences in risk perception and intention to comply when medicines are prescribed for adults or young children. *Psychol Health Med* 2004; 9: 227–234.

35. Gurm HS, Litaker DG. Framing procedural risks to patients: is 99% safe the same risk as a risk of 1 in 100? *Acad Med* 2000; 75: 840–842.

36. McNeil BJ, Pauker SG, Sox HC *et al.* On the elicitation of preferences for alternative therapies. *New Engl J Med* 1982; 306: 1259–1262.

37. Raynor DK, Knapp P, Berry DC. Side effects and patients. In: *Adverse Drug Reactions*, Lee A, ed. London: Pharmaceutical Press, 2006.

38. Knapp P, Gardner P, McMillan B *et al.* The effects of numeracy on the perceived risk of medicine side effects. *Int J Pharm Pract* 2010, 18 (Suppl 2): S23.

39. Keller C, Siegrist M. Effect of risk communication formats on risk perception depending on numeracy. *Med Decis Making* 2009; 29(4): 483–490.

40. Nutbeam D. The evolving concept of health literacy. *Soc Sci Med* 2008; 67: 2072–2078.

41. National Patient Safety Agency. National Reporting and Learning Service. *Quarterly Data Summary Issue 14.* London: NPSA, 2009. http://www.nrls.npsa.nhs.uk/resources/ collections/quarterly-data-summaries/?entryid45=65320

42. Ross S, Bond C, Rothnie H *et al.* What is the scale of prescribing errors committed by junior doctors? A systematic review. *Br J Clin Pharmacol* 2009; 67: 629–640.

43. Garfield S, Barber N, Walley P *et al.* Quality of medication use in primary care: mapping the problem, working to a solution: a systematic review of the literature. *BMC Med* 2009; 7: 50. doi: 10.1186/1741-7015-7-50.

44. Ashcroft D, Morecroft C, Parker D *et al. Patient Safety in Community Pharmacy: Understanding errors and managing risk.* London: RPSGB, 2005. http://www.rpsgb.org/ pdfs/patsafcommph.pdf

45. National Patient Safety Agency. *Risk Assessment Tool for the Preparation and Administration of Injectable Medicines in Clinical Areas.* London: NPSA, 2007. http://www.nrls.npsa.nhs.uk/ resources/?entryid45=59812

46. Reason J. Human error: models and management. *BMJ* 2000; 320: 768–770.

47. Franklin BD, O'Grady K, Donyai P *et al.* The impact of a closed-loop electronic prescribing and administration system on prescribing errors, administration errors and staff time: a before and after study. *Qual Saf Health Care* 2007; 16: 279–284.

48. British Oncology Pharmacists' Association. *Standards for Clinical Pharmacy Verification of Prescriptions for Cancer Medicines.* London: BOPA, 2010. http://www.bopawebsite.org/ tiki page.php?pageName—Position | Statements

49. University of Manchester and National Patient Safety Agency. *Manchester Patient Safety Profile*, 2006. http://www.nrls.npsa.nhs.uk/resources/?entryid45=59796

Useful websites and suggested reading

National Institute for Health Research Service Delivery and Organisation Programme. *Managing Change in the NHS*. London: NIHR. http://www.sdo.nihr.ac.uk/managingchange.html

Department of Health. *Human Resources Change Agents*. London: Department of Health. http://www.dh.gov.uk/en/Publicationsandstatistics/Publications/ PublicationsPolicyAndGuidance/Browsable/DH_5918460

Department of Health. *The NHS Modernisation Agency*. London: Department of Health. http://www.dh.gov.uk/en/Publicationsandstatistics/Publications/AnnualReports/Browsable/ DH_4907637

Institute for Healthcare Improvement (homepage). http://www.ihi.org/ihi

Department of Health. *Building a Safer NHS*. London: Department of Health. http://www.dh. gov.uk/en/Publicationsandstatistics/Publications/PublicationsPolicyAndGuidance/ Browsable/DH_4097460

Department of Health. *Clinical Governance in Community Pharmacy: guidelines on good practice for the NHS*. http://www.dh.gov.uk/en/Publicationsandstatistics/Publications/ PublicationsPolicyAndGuidance/DH_4008717

Krska J. Audit. In: *Pharmaceutical Practice*, 4th edn. Winfield A, Rees J, Smith I, eds. Elsevier, 2009.

National Patient Safety Agency. *Root Cause Analysis Toolkit*. London: NPSA. http://www.nrls. npsa.nhs.uk/resources/collections/root-cause-analysis/

SECTION 3

Improving public health through pharmacy

11

Health education opportunities

Claire Anderson and Alison Blenkinsopp

There are many opportunities for health education in community, hospital and primary care pharmacy practice. This chapter explains health education and health promotion, briefly reviews models of behaviour change and their relevance to health education and summarises the tools used in practical health education, before considering specific health topics of importance to pharmacy.

What is health education?

Health education, as defined by the World Health Organization's health promotion glossary,[1] comprises consciously constructed opportunities for learning which involve some form of communication designed to improve health literacy (see Chapter 10). Although no figures are available, health literacy and numeracy are likely to be low in the UK, as levels of general literacy and numeracy are low. Since people with low health literacy have poorer health than those with adequate health literacy, improving health literacy is an important factor in reducing health inequalities.

As well as improving health literacy, health education includes improving knowledge and developing life skills which are conducive to individual and community health. Health education is not only concerned with the communication of information, but also with fostering the motivation, skills and confidence (self-efficacy) necessary to take action to improve health. It includes the communication of information about the underlying social, economic and environmental conditions impacting on health, as well as individual risk factors, risk behaviours and use of the healthcare system.

Thus health education may involve the communication of information and development of skills which demonstrate the political feasibility and organisational possibilities of various forms of action to address the wider determinants of health (see Chapter 2). In the past, health education was used as a term to encompass these broader actions together with social mobilisation and advocacy. These methods are now covered by the term health promotion and a more narrow definition of health education is used here to emphasise the distinction. Health education is considered to be part of health promotion. Downie, Fyfe and Tannahill[2] developed a model of health promotion comprising three interlinked areas, with health education being one of these (Figure 11.1).

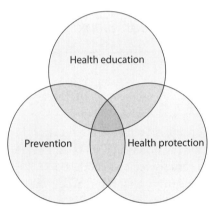

Figure 11.1 Tannahill's model of health promotion. With permission from Downie RS, Fyfe C, Tannahill A. *Health Promotion: Models and values*. Oxford: Oxford University Press, 1990.[2]

Models are useful to help pharmacists (and others) identify their aims in health promotion, the implications of different health promotion strategies, the outcomes of health promotion and their role in health promotion. Models of health promotion are descriptive, not prescriptive. They have been developed to show the scope of existing practice and to chart some of the difficulties with particular ways of working. Downie, Fyfe and Tannahill[2] describe health promotion as comprising efforts to enhance positive health and prevent ill health, through the overlapping spheres of health education, prevention, and health protection.

Aspects of health promotion within the Tannahill model

Health protection deals with regulations and policies and involves governments and other agencies working together to ensure that the social and physical environment is conducive to health. It includes public health measures such as the provision of accessible sports facilities, safe working conditions, for example, a workplace no smoking policy and fiscal measures, excise duty and regulations such as advertising of alcohol and cigarettes (see Chapter 12).

Prevention includes preventive procedures such as screening (see Chapter 13), family planning and immunisation and other preventative action such as the formation of self-help groups. Most health promotion measures are of a preventive nature, being aimed at empowering individuals to adopt healthy lifestyles.

Primary prevention aims at preventing specific diseases developing in individuals. It is directed at healthy individuals, for example, in coronary heart disease, lowering cholesterol by altering diet can reduce the incidence of mortality, and smoking cessation reduces the level of risk to that of non-smokers within about three years of cessation.

Secondary prevention stimulates people to respond to services for early detection and treatment of diseases once they are established, and to ensure that those treated recognise how best they can cooperate to assist with their treatment for management of dyslipidaemia, hypertension, diabetes and weight in coronary heart disease. Interventions directed at depression, social isolation, return to work and other psychosocial issues are examples of secondary prevention.

Tertiary prevention ensures that patients respond effectively where the condition or disease cannot be completely cured. For coronary heart disease, this would seek to reduce the risk of a myocardial infarction or stroke. At one end this may include having a heart transplant but could also mean ensuring that the patient is prescribed appropriate preventive therapy, takes their medicines and adheres to lifestyle advice. This aims to ensure that the individual is helped after diagnosis or treatment to limit the recurrence of the disease, minimise disability and return to active life as soon as possible (see Chapter 13).

Health promotion not only incorporates the three domains of health education, health protection and prevention but also the overlapping areas illustrated in Figure 11.1. Preventive health education includes educational efforts to influence lifestyle in the interests of preventing ill health, as well as efforts to encourage the uptake of preventive services. Preventive health protection addresses policies and regulations of a preventive nature, such as fluoridation of water supplies to prevent dental caries. Health education aimed at health protection involves raising awareness of, and securing support for, positive health protection measures, among the public and policy makers. All three dimensions come together as health education and preventive health protection overlap in efforts to stimulate a social environment conducive to the success of preventive health protection measures, for example, lobbying to ban smoking in work places.

The Beattie health promotion model

A different approach is illustrated by Beattie,[3] who in his structural grid presents a taxonomy of health promotion which attempts to incorporate

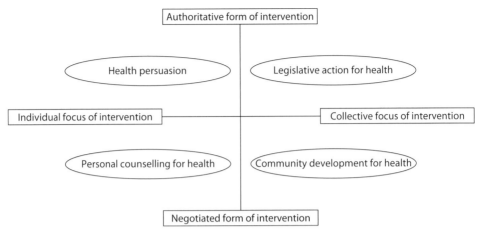

Figure 11.2 Beattie's strategies of health promotion. With permission from reference 3.

the spectrum of activities it includes (Figure 11.2). Beattie's model identifies four discrete areas for health promotion. Activities may be *individual* or *collective*. Interventions may focus on improving the health of individuals, or on improving the health of communities or whole populations. Activities may be *authoritative* or *negotiated*. Authoritative ('top-down') activities are led by practitioners, therefore individuals and communities are encouraged to adopt behaviours that practitioners have decided are good for them. Negotiated ('bottom-up') approaches may be led by lay people themselves, who identify their own health needs, with the practitioner acting as a facilitator.

The grid provides a means of comparing different philosophies of health promoters through analysis of the quadrant where their work originates.

The four approaches identified in Beattie's model are:

- *Health persuasion:* Interventions directed at individuals led by practitioners. This might be considered traditional health education practice, such as providing information to encourage a pregnant woman to stop smoking, and preventive measures, such as screening programmes.
- *Personal counselling:* Client-directed groups in which people are enabled to find their own solutions to their health issues and one-to-one sessions in which the issues discussed are negotiated with the client. Examples are individual or group smoking cessation advice or alcohol counselling.
- *Community development:* Interventions in which groups of people are encouraged to identify and meet their own needs through

education, support or services, with the practitioner acting as a facilitator. For example, a community pharmacist could set up a well man clinic in their local pub.

- *Legislative action for health:* Individual practitioners involved in policy work or lobbying activities, designed to protect the public's health, such as lobbying parliament to increase the price of alcoholic drinks.

Changing behaviour

A large number of psychological models of health-related behaviour have been developed, some of which are useful in health promotion. These can help pharmacists to decide on appropriate interventions which take account of individuals' attitudes towards health issues and their own health. These psychological models focus on individual decision making and have been criticised for ignoring the complexity of health choices and the ways in which they may be constrained by social factors.

The Health Belief Model

The Health Belief Model[4] is used to explain people's health actions. This model suggests that people's behaviour is related to their perceptions of the severity of an illness, their susceptibility to it and the costs and benefits of following a particular course of action. Behaviour may also depend on a trigger, such as a symptom of ill health, the illness of a family member or a friend, or a doctor's advice (Figure 11.3). The premise of the Health Belief Model is that people are basically rational. A limitation of this model is that people may be fearful or in denial and may not always take logical decisions about their own health-related behaviour.

The theory of planned behaviour

The theory of planned behaviour developed by Ajzen[5] is concerned with people's intention to change and their ability to bring about the change. This intention depends on three factors: the individual's attitude towards it, which is in turn determined by their beliefs about the consequences of making the change, subjective norms (the expectations of other people they regard as important), peoples' perceived control over their ability to change and their belief in their own ability to change. The theory of planned behaviour has been applied to a variety of health behaviours including diet, contraceptive use, substance abuse and attending for health screening.

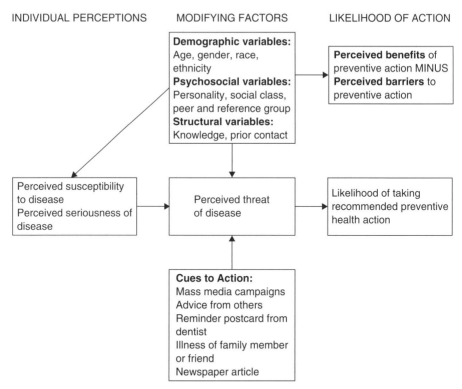

INDIVIDUAL PERCEPTIONS   MODIFYING FACTORS   LIKELIHOOD OF ACTION

Demographic variables:
Age, gender, race, ethnicity
Psychosocial variables:
Personality, social class, peer and reference group
Structural variables:
Knowledge, prior contact

Perceived benefits of preventive action MINUS
Perceived barriers to preventive action

Perceived susceptibility to disease
Perceived seriousness of disease

Perceived threat of disease

Likelihood of taking recommended preventive health action

Cues to Action:
Mass media campaigns
Advice from others
Reminder postcard from dentist
Illness of family member or friend
Newspaper article

Figure 11.3 The Health Belief Model from Becker and Rosenstock[4]
'Milbank Memorial Fund. Reprinted with permission.'

The transtheoretical model

The transtheoretical model[6] suggests that individuals may be at one of a number of stages in a cycle or spiral in relation to making a lifestyle change, illustrated in Figure 11.4. These stages are outlined below.

- *Precontemplation:* clients are not thinking about changing their behaviour; they are not aware that they have a problem and likely to resist any pressure to change.
- *Contemplation:* clients are aware that they have a problem and realise that they must do something about it but have not yet made a commitment to change in the near future.
- *Preparation:* clients begin to make small behavioural changes and make a commitment to take action in the near future.
- *Action:* clients take action to alter their behaviour.
- *Maintenance:* clients continue their efforts towards achieving a permanent change.

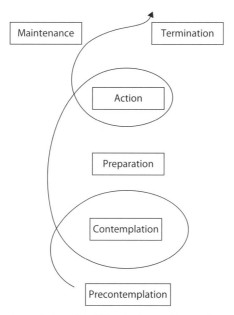

Figure 11.4   The transtheoretical model of lifestyle change. From reference 6.

Precontemplation is the stage at which there is no intention to change the behaviour in the foreseeable future. Many individuals in this stage are unaware or under-aware of their problems or they may have tried to change a number of times before and have become demoralised. For these individuals it is likely to be pressure from others that causes them to seek to change their behaviour and they may do so for as long as pressure is applied, but as soon as this is removed they return to their previous behaviour.

In *contemplation*, people are aware that the problem exists and are seriously thinking about overcoming it in the next six months, but have not made a commitment to take action. Being acutely aware of the pros and cons of changing behaviour and weighing these against each other is an important part of contemplation.

Preparation is a stage that combines intention and behavioural criteria. Individuals in this stage are intending to take action in the next month and often have a plan of action, for example, consulting a health professional or buying a self-help book. They have typically taken some significant action in the past year.

Action is the stage in which individuals modify their behaviour, experiences or their environment, to overcome their problem. Action requires the most overt behavioural change. To be classified as being in the action stage, an individual must have successfully altered their behaviour for a period of from one day to one month.

Maintenance is the stage in which people work to prevent relapse and consolidate the gains attained during action. It is not a static stage but a continuation of change. For most people taking action to modify their behaviour, several attempts are needed before they become long term maintainers. In trying to stop smoking, for example, it can take three or four action attempts before someone becomes a long term maintainer.

Advice giving and interventions

Pharmacy staff can provide information leaflets, while pharmacies can use window displays, touch screens and posters to provide educational messages. PharmacyHealthLink (www.pharmacyhealthlink.org.uk) is a charity that has been working with pharmacy for over 21 years and supplies pharmacists in England with a range of health education materials. A series of cards is available for use with clients in the pharmacy covering physical activity, weight management, diet and nutrition, alcohol, smoking and mental health. However, there are a wide variety of health promotion materials available from many different sources that pharmacists could access and use.

Brief advice and brief interventions are part of the approach to giving opportunistic health advice in a pharmacy, the key distinctions between the two being the time and expertise of pharmacy staff involved, although other factors (such as privacy) might also have an influence. Over the years, three levels of advice giving and interventions have been developed for use in health education: very brief advice (Box 11.1), brief advice and brief interventions.

Box 11.1 *Very brief advice (AAA) to smokers*

This prompt has been developed to enable health professionals to give very brief but clinically effective advice to smokers in as little as 30 seconds using the Ask, Advise, Act approach.[7] It can be used by pharmacists and their staff to focus their conversations and to refer people to other services.

1   *Ask* and record smoking status, ask the client if they are a smoker, ex-smoker or a non-smoker.
2   *Advise* the client of the health benefits of stopping smoking. Tell the client that stopping smoking is the best thing they can do for their health.
3   *Act* on the client' s response.

Build confidence, give information, refer, prescribe.

Brief advice

Brief advice is proactively raising awareness of healthy lifestyle issues and assessing a client's willingness to engage in further discussion about them. It is usually given opportunistically and is usually linked to the supply of a medicine, product or service requested by the client visiting the pharmacy. It should normally take no more than three minutes and follow this structure:

- *Listen* – to the client's needs or concerns.
- *Observe* – for signs of health-related or lifestyle issues, e.g. nicotine-stained fingers.
- *Ask* – raise issues in a non-threatening manner using indirect questions to start with. Examples of indirect questions include: 'Have you seen our promotion/advertisement for a healthy lifestyle consultation?'; 'We are offering our customers the opportunity to check if their weight is within the healthy range – would you like any advice or help with this?'
- *Assess* – the client's response. Do they appear willing to engage in further discussion on this topic?
- *Advise* – if the client is interested then give general health advice or lead into specific brief interventions as appropriate. But if the client is not keen to have further discussions then they should be told they can come back and ask any questions, or look through the health information available in the pharmacy.
- *Record* – the outcome. Did this discussion entail brief advice only or did it lead to an intervention? Was the person particularly sensitive to this issue? If so, why? Did you refer or advise the person to follow up? If yes, where and when?

Brief interventions

Brief interventions occur when a client responds positively to proactive brief advice or specifically asks for help with a health-related issue. The model for giving brief interventions in a pharmacy setting[7] has been adapted from NICE guidance for smoking cessation.[8] It should typically take up to 30 minutes and include:

- giving simple opportunistic advice to change
- assessing a client's commitment to change
- supplying self-help materials or resources
- offering pharmacotherapy and behavioural support as appropriate
- providing specialist support (if suitably trained) or refer or 'signpost' to specialist support

- offering a follow-up appointment if appropriate
- recording the outcome of discussion.

An offer of, or provision of or referral to, specialist behavioural support with or without pharmacotherapy should only occur when the client concerned has shown sufficient interest or motivation in making healthy lifestyle choices. The particular intervention that is provided will depend on a number of factors, including the individual's willingness to follow the advice, how acceptable they find the intervention on offer and the previous ways they have tried to change their behaviour.

Motivational interviewing is also a potentially useful approach advocated by many pharmacy organisations in different countries. It is a type of communication technique designed to help an individual identify their own goals, then work towards achieving them. This has the theoretical advantage of ensuring ownership of the goals by the client, since they are lead towards drawing their own conclusions as to what these should be, rather than goals being suggested by the pharmacist. Motivational interviewing complements the transtheoretical model of change (see page 182) and seeks to create a collaborative approach between client and health professional. This enables the client to clarify their strengths and aspirations, evoke motivations for changing behaviour and maintain control over changes they decide to make. Motivational interviewing has been used to improve adherence to medication in a variety of settings and has been shown to be feasible in UK community pharmacy settings in relation to alcohol and drug misuse.

Practical health education

The potential contribution of pharmacy to improve the health of the public has long been recognised, and even more so with increasing emphasis on the prevention of ill health (see Chapter 1). Although pharmacists in all health sectors have many opportunities to engage in health education activities, much of the research evidence has been obtained from evaluation of community pharmacy activities. Through the 2005 community pharmacy contract for England and Wales, public health for the first time became part of the everyday work of the pharmacy. Pharmacists are expected to proactively participate in national/local campaigns, by promoting public health messages to pharmacy users during specific targeted campaign periods. All pharmacies are required to provide prescription-linked brief advice on issues of public health concern to those who have diabetes or are at risk of coronary heart disease, especially those with high blood pressure or who smoke or are overweight and to participate in up to six local health campaigns each year. Furthermore community pharmacies can provide enhanced services, commissioned and funded locally by PCTs to meet local needs. Examples include smoking cessation, free emergency hormonal contraception, screening for and treatment of *Chlamydia* infection and vascular risk check and management. Similar core services are provided by community pharmacies in Scotland, but there are nationally specified services for supporting smoking cessation and a sexual health service that provides free emergency hormonal contraception and *Chlamydia* testing and treatment.

We have completed three structured reviews of the international peer reviewed literature on community pharmacy's contribution to improving the public's health covering the periods 1990–2001 and 2001–2004 and 2004–7.[9–12] These showed there was good evidence from randomised controlled trials of the effectiveness of community pharmacy services in some areas (lipid management, smoking cessation) and some evidence in other areas. However, the number of robust evaluations was small and raised issues about the strength of the evidence base for community pharmacy interventions in general. The evidence is summarised here.

Smoking cessation

Background

Smoking is the single greatest cause of preventable morbidity and premature deaths in England, with half a million hospital admissions among adults aged over 35 attributed to smoking. Smoking-related diseases are currently estimated to cost the NHS around £1.5 billion a year. Stop smoking services are one of the most cost-effective of all NHS health interventions and it is one of the most frequently commissioned local enhanced services from community pharmacies in England.

Smoking is the main reason for the gap in life expectancy between rich and poor with smoking being responsible, in men, for over half the excess risk of premature death between social classes. It is also implicated in cancer, coronary heart disease, stroke and other circulatory diseases, respiratory disease, stomach and duodenal ulcers, erectile dysfunction and infertility, osteoporosis, cataracts, age-related macular degeneration and periodontitis.

Women who smoke during pregnancy have a much higher risk of miscarriage, and smoking can lead to complications in pregnancy and labour. Babies born to women who smoke tend to be lighter, which can increase the risk of death and disease in childhood. Smoking in pregnancy increases infant mortality by about 40%. Passive smoking can exacerbate respiratory symp toms among non-smokers and has also been linked to cot deaths and respiratory diseases in babies and in the longer term increases the risk of lung cancer, heart disease and stroke.

Opportunities for pharmacy intervention

Opportunistic advice about stopping smoking can be given by community pharmacists and their staff when signs of smoking are observed, e.g. nicotine-stained fingers, buying smoker's toothpaste and repeated requests for cough remedies. More overt requests about stopping smoking and to purchase nicotine replacement therapy also present opportunities for intervention. Some pharmacists have been trained as smoking cessation counsellors and appropriately trained pharmacy staff can also be involved in interventions, particularly in checking people's smoking status and giving very brief advice.

Combining behavioural support with pharmacotherapy increases a smoker's chance of successfully stopping by up to four times. Clients who wish to stop smoking should be given the optimum chance of success in any quit attempt. Nicotine replacement therapy is available for sale in pharmacies in the UK and many other countries. In the UK it can also be supplied on the NHS or privately rather than sold, by using patient group directions (PGDs). (A patient group direction is a group prescribing protocol that provides the legal authority for suitably trained pharmacists or nurses to supply a prescription only medicine to requesting clients, where they can benefit patient care without compromising safety.) PGDs can also be used to facilitate the provision of varenicline and bupropion. Bupropion should only be provided to a smoker who commits to a target stop date, while varenicline should normally only be supplied as part of a programme of behavioural smoking cessation support.[8] Varenicline is reported to be associated with some serious adverse drug reactions, including suicidal thoughts and behaviour; therefore, if used in patients with a history of psychiatric illness, they should be monitored closely. A comparison of the effectiveness of different interventions and products is shown in Table 11.1.

Table 11.1 Comparison of quit rates using drugs recommended by NICE as cost-effective for supporting smoking cessation

	Four-week quit rates (%)			
	No medication	NRT	Bupropion	Varenicline
No support	16	25	28	37
Individual behavioural support	22	37	39	52
Group behavioural support	32	50	55	74

From NHS stop smoking services. Service and monitoring guidance 2009/10.
NRT = nicotine replacement therapy.

Evidence

There is strong evidence from randomised controlled trials that trained pharmacists providing brief advice and brief interventions are effective in smoking cessation. Community pharmacy-based smoking cessation services, run by trained pharmacists and their staff have been shown to be effective and cost-effective. There is also some evidence of effectiveness of the involvement of pharmacists in smoking cessation in hospital pharmacy and prison settings and of the feasibility of using a computer programme as the basis for a community pharmacy-based smoking cessation service.[12]

Training, especially in behaviour change methods (see page 181), has been found to be essential to the success of pharmacy smoking cessation services. Without training, pharmacists are more likely to take a reactive rather than proactive approach and to simply respond to smokers' requests for advice rather than to proactively initiate conversations about smoking. There is potential benefit to be gained from a whole staff approach in community pharmacy, although there are no comparative data for when pharmacists alone have provided the service.

Emergency hormonal contraception

Background

In England, the rate of conception in women aged 15 to 17 increased in 2007 for the first time in several years, to 41.9 conceptions per 1000 women. There was also a rise in the under-16 conception rate to 8.3 per 1000 girls aged 13–15. This amounted to an estimated 8196 conceptions to girls aged under 16 in 2007. However, both the under-16 and under-18 abortion rates in 2008 were lower than 2007 rates. The UK still has the highest rate of teenage pregnancy in Europe, but the issue is of international concern.

National sexual health strategies have been developed in all countries of the UK, which include reducing under-18 conceptions as a specific target for modification. Unintended pregnancies among teenagers are most common in girls from poor backgrounds and are associated with poor social, economic and health outcomes for both mother and infant.

Opportunities for pharmacy intervention

UK community pharmacy involvement with contraception began in the 1980s, with the Family Planning Association championing pharmacies as a readily accessible location for advice. During the past decade the increasing percentage of community pharmacies with consultation facilities has improved the level of privacy and paved the way for extended services. Community pharmacy supply of levonorgestrel emergency hormonal contraception (EHC) became widespread in the UK after two important changes.

The first, in 2000, led by innovative primary care organisations, was the introduction of a service to supply EHC when appropriate to clients in line with the requirements of a locally agreed PGD (see page 188). The second was the deregulation of the EHC product containing levonorgestrel in 2001 to make it available over the counter under the control of pharmacists, now also similarly available in many other countries. These two developments widened access to EHC, although there are some differences between them. Supply through a PGD provides the prescribable product free of charge at NHS expense, usually for women up to 24 years, as if on a NHS prescription, but can also be supplied to girls under 16, depending on the conditions laid down by the PGD. The over-the-counter product is only available for sale to women over 16 years of age. The RPSGB has produced practice guidance on the supply of EHC.[13]

Pharmacies are expected to offer a user friendly, non-judgemental, client centred and confidential service. Pharmacists who supply EHC via PGD must have completed accredited training, which includes child protection training. They should be aware of local networks for community contraceptive services, so that women who need to see a doctor can be referred on rapidly. Women unable to receive EHC because they are excluded through the PGD criteria must be referred as soon as possible to another local service that will be able to assist them, such as a GP or community contraception service. If the exclusion is only because of administrative reasons, such as age restriction, rather than clinical reasons, clients can be invited to purchase the pharmacy medicine product instead.

Pharmacists are also expected to provide support and advice to women accessing the service, including advice on the avoidance of pregnancy and sexually transmitted infections (STIs) through safer sex and condom use, advice on the use of regular contraceptive methods and provide onward signposting to services that provide long term contraceptive methods and diagnosis and management of STIs. The ideal public health goal should be to reduce unprotected sexual intercourse and hence reliance on EHC, by persuading women to change their behaviour.

Evidence

There is considerable evidence for this service to be provided from pharmacies.[12] One UK study, following the deregulation of EHC, showed a subsequent decrease in requests for EHC in accident and emergency departments. Training has been shown to improve pharmacists' performance in supply of EHC in accordance with protocols and mystery shopping indicated that pharmacists' supply is according to protocols in most cases.

Pharmacists have been shown to be very satisfied with delivering EHC services and view them as a way to improve their role in patient-focused care. Some pharmacists have concerns about the potential for repeated use of EHC and the possible effect of easier access to EHC, on the incidence of STIs. Making EHC available over the counter did not change the level of use, but did change where women obtained it from, with more women using pharmacies as the source. A large, American trial of the provision of EHC in advance found no increase in risky sexual behaviour and no significant reduction in the number of pregnancies. No differences were observed in use of regular contraception or in risky sexual behaviour by women obtaining EHC from pharmacies, and adolescents aged younger than 16 years behaved no differently in response to increased access to EHC from other age groups.

In most studies pharmacy services were highly rated by women. Women had some concerns about confidentiality and privacy, particularly younger women. In general, the way in which services are configured affects their use, with women preferring services that give them privacy while treating them in a sympathetic and non-judgemental manner. It is worth noting that many of the studies were conducted prior to the increase in availability of consultation areas in pharmacies; most UK pharmacies now have such an area. Some concerns were also reported by service users about the appropriateness and timeliness of additional and unsolicited information and advice from pharmacists about future contraceptive use and STIs. Pharmacists need training to provide this advice in an appropriate manner.

Contraception

A number of pharmacists in England have recently begun to provide oral contraceptive services. The first NHS community pharmacy service for the initiation and supply of combined oral contraception and progesterone-only contraception was introduced in 2008. Further research is needed to evaluate these emerging models of possible future sexual health services in community pharmacies in the UK. There are a number of schemes around the country where pharmacists, like family planning centres, are able to provide free condoms (see Box 11.2).

Box 11.2 *Supply of free condoms*

Pharmacists in Nottingham city are involved in the c-card scheme, a service for young people aged 13–24 years, where they can get free condoms, lubricants and advice about sex and relationships (www.ccardnottingham.co.uk). The card allows the young person to approach the pharmacy staff without having to give an embarrassing explanation of why they are there. The c-card logo is displayed in the pharmacy window. Clients register at a number of different agencies then they can take their c-card to a participating pharmacy to receive the service.

Sexually transmitted infections

Background

Chlamydia is the most common sexually transmitted infection (STI) in the UK, affecting as many as one in ten sexually active young men and women, with the highest prevalence in those under 25 years of age. Untreated infection can have serious long term consequences, particularly for women. It can lead to pelvic inflammatory disease, ectopic pregnancy and tubal factor infertility. Since many infections are asymptomatic, a large proportion of people are unaware they are infected, although infection can be diagnosed easily and effectively treated.

The DoH in England has implemented a national *Chlamydia* screening programme, enabling free testing for 16–24 year olds. The objective of the programme is to control *Chlamydia* through the early detection and treatment of asymptomatic infection, preventing the development of sequelae and reducing onward transmission of the disease. An opportunistic approach is used, involving a diverse combination of healthcare and non-healthcare screening venues, plus voluntary and business sectors. Community pharmacies have become an important part of this programme.

Opportunities for pharmacy intervention

Pharmacies that deliver the service provide *Chlamydia* screening kits to sexually active males and females under the age of 25; for example, when purchasing condoms, dispensing oral contraceptive pills and supplying EHC, in agreement with the local *Chlamydia* screening office. A complementary private *Chlamydia* screening service, via sales of test kits, operates in parallel for those who do not have access to the service and for over 25s. Advice on how to use the kit, how to return it for testing and what will happen following completion of the test is given.

Pharmacists may also inform people of their test results, undertake contact tracing and offer treatment in line with the requirements of a locally agreed PGD.

The pharmacist ensures that azithromycin or doxycycline (second line treatment) is suitable for the client, informs them of the need for complete abstinence from sexual contact until treatment for both the client and partner is completed and provide further advice about the possible risks of other STIs.

Evidence

The feasibility of providing *Chlamydia* screening through community pharmacies has been demonstrated by pilot studies in the UK and the Netherlands.[12] The service appeared to increase access to testing among those who would not otherwise have been tested and could potentially reduce demand from other sexual health services (Box 11.3). Further work is

> ***Box 11.3*** *Chlamydia screening in pharmacies*
>
> Boots ran a two-year *Chlamydia* screening and treatment pilot on behalf of the DoH as part of the national *Chlamydia* screening programme in England. This aimed to assess pharmacies as an access point for *Chlamydia* testing and treatment by offering free testing kits to 16–24 year olds at 216 Boots pharmacies in London. In total, 21 793 pharmacy screens were undertaken between November 2005 and 30 June 2007. Around 80% of the screens (19 909) resulted in a conclusive positive or negative test result and the remainder were inconclusive. The overall positivity rate in this group was 8% (7% females; 10% males) which is lower than the 10.1% overall positivity rate reported in the programme as a whole for this period. However, more men accessed the Boots programme than other providers; male users comprised 21% of all pharmacy users.

required to encourage uptake by young men and in improving confidentiality at the pharmacy counter. A report on the overall national *Chlamydia* screening programme identified that it was not meeting its objectives, in particular, only 88% of those who tested positive had received treatment, partner notification rates were lower than necessary and only 60% of young people had received advice on contraception and safer sex.

Research in sexual health has emanated from a wide range of countries and the role of the community pharmacist in sexual health is developing worldwide. *Choosing Health through Pharmacy*[14] stated that there was evidence that community pharmacy could provide sexual health services and indicated that the government would like pharmacy to do more. Access to training that incorporates and encourages networking with other local service providers is likely to be crucial in increasing pharmacists' confidence in dealing with these issues appropriately and effectively.

Osteoporosis risk assessment/prevention

Background

Osteoporosis is a condition in which the density and quality of bone is reduced, increasing the risk of fracture. It affects around one in three women and one in five men globally. Bone mineral density, assessed by dual-energy X-ray absorptiometry (DXA) is the gold standard for the diagnosis of osteoporosis. However, it is possible to assess risk, since there is a wide range of factors which increase the likelihood of developing the condition, enabling the selection of people who should receive DXA scanning for confirmation of diagnosis. Skeletal and non-skeletal risk factors can be combined to identify those at highest risk of fracture, using case-finding strategies. Risk factors are listed in Box 11.4.

Box 11.4 *Risk factors for osteoporosis*

Modifiable factors

Cigarette smoking

Excessive alcohol consumption

Low body mass index

Low dietary calcium intake

Vitamin D deficiency

Prolonged immobilisation – little or no physical activity

Visual impairment

Frequent falls

Non-modifiable factors

Female gender

Premature menopause

Primary or secondary amenorrhoea

Primary and secondary hypogonadism in men

Age 60 or over

Asian or Caucasian race

Previous fragility fracture

Family history of hip fracture

Low bone mineral density

High bone turnover

Neuromuscular disorders

Long term steroid therapy

Rheumatoid arthritis

Risk factors can provide additional information on the risk of fracture independently of measuring bone mineral density. In areas or countries with limited or no access to densitometry, clinical risk factors can be used for risk assessment.

Opportunities for pharmacy intervention

Pharmacists can identify patients at potential risk through case-searching using patient medication records. These could include patients taking drugs that indicate one of the conditions listed in Box 11.4 as well as those at risk of falls because of adverse effects of medicines, such as postural hypotension or drowsiness. Customers purchasing calcium and vitamin D tablets may benefit from screening.

Evidence

Osteoporosis services such as fracture risk assessment, falls prevention and a risk management service for people taking long term oral cortico-steroids have been successfully provided from community pharmacies and are well received. They have identified women at different levels of fracture risk. Overall the evidence shows that community pharmacy-based bone health assessments can identify people who need to be referred for further medical investigation.[12] There is also some evidence that advice given to women identified to be at lower risk may result in increased dietary intake of calcium and increased exercise.

Oral health

Background

Although there has been a decline in dental caries in developed countries over the past 20 years, largely as a result of effective use of fluorides, changes in lifestyles and self care measures, it is still a major health problem in most industrialised countries, affecting 60–90% of school-age children and nearly 100% of adults. Oral cancer affects around 4900 people every year in the UK. It is more common in men than women and the vast majority of cases occur in people aged over 50. Smoking is the largest single risk factor for oral cancer and contributes to over 90% of cases as well as causing periodontal disease and premature tooth loss. Alcohol use is also a risk factor.

Opportunities for pharmacy intervention

Pharmacists have numerous opportunities to provide education about oral health. They sell toothbrushes, toothpaste and mouth washes and supply medicines for children, which should generally be sugar free. Pharmacies are also a frequent source of advice on dental pain, mouth ulcers and other oral health issues. However, there is very little evidence and no recent evidence on the contribution of community pharmacy to improving oral health.[11] Most pharmacists have reported receiving little or no training relating to oral health education.

Weight management

Background

Obesity is recognised as a major threat to current and future health and globally its incidence has increased markedly during recent years (see Chapter 2). Reducing levels of obesity is a key priority in the UK.

Opportunities for pharmacy intervention

Pharmacists may encounter people who are wishing to lose weight frequently, since many pharmacies have installed machines to measure weight, height and BMI. In addition, they currently are the major retail source of over-the-counter weight loss products.[15] Although these in general lack evidence of efficacy, pharmacists could use the opportunity to promote more effective weight management programmes.

Evidence

Few published studies have evaluated community pharmacy weight-management services. In published studies the interventions were generally fairly intensive in terms of pharmacist input but showed weight loss of up to 5 kg. None of the studies to date have included an economic evaluation of the service provided. Currently the evidence for weight management might best be summed up as 'promising and in need of further study'.[12] Some PCTs are however, commissioning weight management services from community pharmacies. One of the first of these was in Coventry, where the first 34 clients who completed 10 follow-up visits to their pharmacy lost an average of around 4 kg (see Box 3.4, page 37).

Physical activity

Background

The potential benefits to health that could result from increased physical activity are huge. If everyone adopted the recommended levels of physical activity, the overall gain in health would be: nearly a third of all coronary heart disease incidence avoided, a quarter of strokes avoided, nearly a quarter of non-insulin dependent diabetes in over 45 year olds avoided, and just over half the hip fractures in over 45 year olds avoided.

Opportunities for pharmacy intervention

The informal atmosphere of the pharmacy together with the regular contact with the public and the provision of services such as vascular and diabetes screening make the pharmacy an excellent setting for this sort of health education. Pharmacists come into contact with many people who could benefit from increased physical activity and in addition can target specific groups of patients using patient medication records. Local campaigns encouraging the public to get advice on physical activity from community pharmacies offer the chance to raise awareness of the pharmacist's role and increase customer loyalty.

Evidence

There is very little evidence on the effectiveness of pharmacy-based interventions to increase physical activity. A randomised controlled trial in one community pharmacy tested an intervention comprising an individualised plan for action in relation to diet, physical activity, obesity and alcohol intake. Blood pressure control improved significantly in the intervention group. However, it is difficult to assess the impact of the non-drug aspect of the intervention as the pharmacists also identified and made recommendations about drug-related problems.[12]

Alcohol intake

Background

Alcohol misuse is a major public health concern. One in four adults in the UK drink above the recommended limits and binge drinking is on the increase. There are many health risks associated with drinking too much alcohol, including anxiety, sexual difficulties such as impotence, slowed breathing and heartbeat, impaired judgement leading to accidents and injuries, loss of consciousness, suffocation through choking on your own vomit and potentially fatal alcohol poisoning. The long term health risks include coronary heart disease, liver disease and psychoses (see Chapter 2).

Opportunities for pharmacy interventions

Screening using a short structured questionnaire, followed by brief interventions, is effective in reducing alcohol consumption and can be successfully delivered in a primary care setting. Delivery of the intervention generally comprises a short verbal/counselling session of 5–10 minutes, written information to take away, and occasionally a diary to record alcohol intake. These interventions are suitable for use in pharmacies, but it is important to ensure effective ways of approaching clients appropriate to pharmacies are used. Opportunities present when customers purchase hangover cures, products for upset stomach or during screening for cardiovascular disease, to name a few.

Evidence

There has been little published evaluation of pharmacy involvement in the provision of services for alcohol misuse.[16] Three small, proof-of-concept studies have demonstrated that screening for excessive alcohol consumption can be delivered in community pharmacies and can be followed by the delivery of brief interventions to clients identified as harmful or hazardous drinkers. Two of the studies reported non-significant reductions in alcohol consumption following brief interventions by pharmacists. The third study recorded the number of people screened and interventions delivered, without follow up. The proportion of pharmacy customers identified as having hazardous or harmful drinking behaviour ranged from 30–53%. Larger studies are needed to generate more definitive evidence.

In the meantime some PCTs are commissioning services from community pharmacies (Box 11.5).

Box 11.5 *Alcohol screening and brief interventions*

Pharmacies in Wirral, Merseyside have been contracted to deliver a coordinated alcohol identification, screening and brief intervention programme as part of the Wirral Alcohol Harm Reduction Strategy 2007–2010. In the programme, pharmacists raise public awareness about alcohol usage, safe drinking limits and calculation of units per drink. In the first year, over 2100 clients were screened.

Training and practical experience has enabled pharmacy staff to engage their customers in a conversation about alcohol. An easy start to the conversation is with someone waiting for a prescription for a medicine that interacts with alcohol. The significant change is that staff have become used to introducing the subject with customers who are buying medicines or making other purchases in a non-intrusive way. Once the interaction has been begun a questionnaire is used to assess drinking habits and using a scoring system, people are offered information, behavioural change techniques or referral to a specialist service. The 10-question questionnaire allocates a points total indicating whether the client is at low risk, hazardous, harmful or dependent levels of drinking. Follow up is at 8 and 52 weeks. Experience has shown that many of the people screened did not understand how many units of alcohol were contained in different drinks and thus were sometimes shocked to find out their weekly intake.

Mental health

Background

Mental health is a vital component of overall health and improving public mental health is increasingly recognised as important. Depression is a major public health problem, and mental ill health is the highest cause of disability worldwide. In England, mental illness results not only in major expense to the NHS but also reduced quality of life and lost output through time off work, and can also have significant impact on physical health. Recently a new strategy document has been produced by the DoH, which encourages greater promotion of mental health.[17]

Opportunities for pharmacy interventions

There are simple screening tools available for identifying mental health problems that could be used in pharmacies; however, little has been done to explore this possibility. Social prescribing is increasingly receiving attention as an alternative to the use of drugs for patients with mild depression and anxiety and could easily be promoted by pharmacy staff. Social prescribing is non-medical support which could include arts and creative activities, volunteering, help with financial problems, exercise programmes and many other actions. There is evidence that social prescribing can be effective in helping people with mild to moderate depression and anxiety and enables a proactive approach to mental health promotion.

Pharmacies could use posters, leaflets and window displays to promote mental health awareness and staff are ideally placed to provide health education advice to people purchasing non-prescription medicines for sleep disorders, anxiety or depression. Pharmacists could also advise clients and their carers when dispensing prescriptions for medicines used in treating mental illness. At present mental health education is an area which has not been researched in pharmacy.

Healthy-living pharmacies

As we look to the future it is likely that more healthy-living pharmacies will be developed. The pharmacy White Paper, *Building on Strengths, Delivering the Future*,[18] sets out a vision for pharmacy service development in the future. This includes pharmacies as centres promoting and supporting healthy living and health literacy, offering patients and the public healthy-lifestyle advice and support for self care and a range of pressing public health concerns. These include influenza, treating minor ailments and expanding and improving the range of clinical services to people, in particular those with long term conditions, through routine monitoring, screening and support in making the best use of their medicines.

References

1. World Health Organization. *Health Promotion Glossary*. http://www.who.int/healthpromotion/about/HPG/en/ (accessed 9 February 10).
2. Downie RS, Fyfe C, Tannahill A. *Health Promotion: Models and values*. Oxford: Oxford University Press, 1990.
3. Beattie A. Knowledge and control in health promotion. In: Gabe J, Calman M, Bury M. *Sociology of the Health Service*. London: Routledge Kegan and Paul, 1990.
4. Rosenstock IM (1966). Why people use health services. *Milbank Mem Fund Q* 44: 94–124, 1990.
5. Ajzen I. The theory of planned behaviour. *Organ Behav Hum Decis Process* 1991; 50(2): 179–211.
6. Prochaska J, Diclimente C. *Transtheoretical Therapy: Towards a More Integrative Model of Change*. Homewood, Illinois: Dow Jones and Irwin, 1982.
7. PharmacyHealthLink. *Brief Advice versus Brief Interventions*. http://www.pharmacymeetspublichealth.org.uk/pdf/10389%20BA%20vers%20BI%20doc-a.pdf (accessed 9 February 2010).

8. National Institute of Health and Clinical Excellence. *Brief Interventions and Referral for Smoking Cessation*. London: NICE, 2006. http://www.nice.org.uk/PHI001 (accessed 9 February 2010).

9. Anderson C, Blenkinsopp A, Armstrong M. *Report 5. The Contribution of Pharmacy to Improving the Public's Health: Evidence from the peer-reviewed literature 2001–2004*. London: PharmacyHealthLink and RPSGB. http://www.phlink.org.uk/?q=evidence_base_reports (accessed 9 February 2010).

10. Anderson C, Blenkinsopp A, Armstrong M. *Report 6. The Contribution of Community Pharmacy to Improving the Public's Health: Literature review update 2004–2007. A management summary of evidence published in peer-reviewed journals over the past 3 years*. PharmacyHealthLink and RPSGB, 2008. http://www.phlink.org.uk/?q=evidence_base_reports (accessed 9 February 2010).

11. Anderson C, Blenkinsopp A, Armstrong M. *Report 1. The Contribution of Community Pharmacy to Improving the Public's Health: Evidence from the peer reviewed literature 1990–2001*. London: PharmacyHealthLink and RPSGB, 2003. http://www.phlink.org.uk/?q=evidence_base_reports (accessed 9 February 2010).

12. Anderson C, Blenkinsopp A, Armstrong M. *Report 7. The Contribution of Community Pharmacy to Improving the Public's Health: Summary report of the literature review 1990–2007*. London: PharmacyHealthLink and RPSGB, 2009. http://www.phlink.org.uk/?q=evidence_base_reports (accessed 9 February 2010).

13. Royal Pharmaceutical Society of Great Britain. *Practice Guidance on the Supply of Emergency Hormonal Contraception as a Pharmacy Medicine*. London: RPSGB, 2004. http://www.rpsgb.org.uk/pdfs/ehcguid.pdf (accessed 9 February 2010).

14. Department of Health. *Choosing Health through Pharmacy: A programme for pharmaceutical public health 2005–2015*. London: TSO 2005. http://www.dh.gov.uk/dr_consum_dh/groups/dh_digitalassets/@dh/@en/documents/digitalasset/dh_4107496.pdf (accessed 9 February 2010).

15. Krska J, Lovelady C, Connolly D *et al*. Weight management services in community pharmacy: identifying opportunities. *Int J Pharm Pract* 2010 (in press).

16. Watson MC, Blenkinsopp A. The feasibility of providing community pharmacy based services for alcohol misuse: a literature review. *Int J Pharm Prac* 2009; 17(4): 199–205.

17. HM Government. *New Horizons: A shared vision for mental health*. London: Department of Health, 2009. http://newhorizons.dh.gov.uk/Resources/reports/New-Horizons/index.aspx.

18. Department of Health. *Building on Strengths: Delivering the future*. London: TSO, 2010. http://www.dh.gov.uk/en/News/Recentstories/DH_097701 (accessed 9 February 2010).

12

Health protection

Adam J Mackridge

Health protection seeks to care for a population (or a sub-set of the population, e.g. those aged over 65 years) through containing communicable diseases (preventing them spreading) and minimising harm caused by potential threats to health. It focuses on the population rather than individuals, seeking to protect the health of everyone within a population, rather than treating persons suffering from ill health. For example, identifying a patient with tuberculosis requires notification (see Chapter 1) because of the need to minimise the spread of this disease among the wider population. The patient may be segregated from other patients and infection control measures put in place.

In most developed countries, a government organisation exists, with the remit of protecting the community against infectious disease and other dangers to health, preventing the spread of infectious disease, and providing assistance to other people and agencies. In the UK this is currently the Health Protection Agency (HPA). This body is responsible for identifying and responding to health hazards or emergencies in relation to communicable diseases and other hazards to health. To identify emerging risks to public health and track the impact of health protection measures, it is important to maintain accurate data. This is particularly true for communicable diseases and the HPA Centre for Infections is currently responsible for collating data on notifiable diseases that pose a risk to public health. These data are used to advise governments on appropriate action to respond to specific threats to the population, such as the swine flu (H1N1 virus strain) pandemic in 2009 (see page 64 and Box 12.4). Further information on surveillance processes is given in Chapter 4.

As experts on the manufacture and use of medicines, pharmacists have traditionally had a role in health protection by ensuring the safe production and supply of medicines. However, owing to developments in both the role of the pharmacist – towards a more general health expert – and approaches to handling issues around substance use, pharmacists have increasingly had wider health protection roles, encompassing a range of activities in all sectors. Pharmacists are now routinely involved at a strategic level, for example, the development of antibiotic formularies and safe storage policies or planning responses to specific health issues, and at an individual level in delivery of health protection interventions such as provision of needles and syringes to drug users, or facilitating the safe disposal of unwanted medicines.

This chapter explores three key elements of health protection where pharmacists have a role: protecting against the potential harms caused by medicines; substance use; and communicable diseases.

Protecting against the potential harms caused by medicines

Licensing of medicines

In most countries, there is some degree of control over the manufacture and supply of medicinal products (substances used for treatment, diagnosis or prevention of a disease) to protect against harm caused by poor quality products or inappropriate use. In the UK, legislation attempting to protect the public in this way was first introduced in the 16th century, initially to prevent adulteration or contamination of drugs and eventually limiting supply routes to health professionals. During the early stages of this process, medicines were often included in legislation along with foods or poisons. More modern approaches to regulating medicines began to be implemented in Europe in the 1960s. This began with a directive, issued by the European Economic Community in 1965, that placed controls on the sale and supply of medicines in member states. In the UK, this directive was incorporated into the Medicines Act (1968) and the Misuse of Drugs Act (1971), which also brought other legislation relating to medicines together for the first time. Following this, medicines were clearly identified as different from other items of commerce, reflecting their unique attributes of potential for doing good and also for causing harm, with regulation (through licensing) of manufacture, import, advertising, sale and supply. These acts have since been extensively added to and amended and, in some aspects, superseded by further European Community directives, making it likely that they will be replaced entirely by new legislation in future.

A key international incident involving thalidomide, a drug used in the treatment of morning sickness in pregnant women, also highlighted the need for better regulation of medicines in the 1960s. At the time, requirements for testing of medicines prior to sale were limited and thalidomide was used widely in many countries, with both patients and health professionals unaware of its potential for teratogenicity. Only after thousands of babies were born with physical deformities was the cause traced to the drug and its use in pregnant women ceased. Through the various regulatory frameworks now in place throughout the world, tragedies such as this are now considerably less likely to occur, as drugs are considered on safety, quality and efficacy prior to being granted a licence for sale. In the UK, such licences are referred to as marketing authorisations and are granted and administered by the Medicines and Healthcare products Regulatory Agency (MHRA).

This body reviews evidence on new and current medicines and balances the risk of use in patients and to the wider public against the benefits to patients and public health. The Commission on Human Medicines (formerly Committee on Safety of Medicines), which traces its origins back to the thalidomide tragedy, advises the MHRA. Medicines licensing is undertaken by the Food and Drug Administration in the USA, the Therapeutic Goods Administration in Australia and the European Medicines Agency (EMA) in the European Union (EU). The EMA differs from the other agencies in that it acts as a centralised regulatory agency for the EU, with powers to grant authorisations for medicines in all member states, without the need for approval from the respective agencies within each state. At present, manufacturers can choose whether to approach the regulatory body in each member state of the EU or to apply for blanket approval from the EMA. All these bodies also have responsibilities for ensuring that medicines manufactured in their respective jurisdictions meet rigorous standards in terms of ingredients used, manufacturing processes and quality control and extensive guidance on good manufacturing practice has been issued.

In the UK, the Medicines Act sets out three levels of availability for medicines: general availability (general sales list; GSL medicines); sale under the supervision of a pharmacist (pharmacy; P medicines); and sale or supply in response to a prescription from an appropriate practitioner (prescription-only medicine; POM). When marketing authorisations are granted for new medicines, they are usually placed in the POM category initially until further safety data are available from use in the wider population. During initial use of newly licensed medicines, post-marketing surveillance is employed to evaluate safety in a wider population. This includes review of the safety of medicines in population subgroups, such as the elderly, and in the UK data is gathered through the Yellow Card Scheme. Should a drug demonstrate a good safety profile during the post marketing surveillance phase, further applications for reclassification to P, and eventually GSL, may then be accepted. Further information on the Yellow Card Scheme and post-marketing surveillance is given in Chapter 14.

Moving medicines to categories with fewer controls makes them more accessible to the population, supporting self care. This is now a common occurrence in the UK and increasing numbers of applications have been made in recent years to transfer medicines from POM to P or GSL status.

Applications are reviewed by regulatory bodies on the basis of the potential risks posed to health of individuals and the wider population. Thus even where a drug poses little risk to individuals using it, applications for reclassification may be refused on the basis of risks to the population – for example, antibiotic products with a significant risk of resistance (see page 216).

In many other countries, there are fewer restrictions on the availability of medicines and pharmacies may be the main supplier of all medicines through purchase, rather than against prescription (see Chapter 5). In this situation, as well as when medicines are deliberately classified for self care, pharmacists' activities provide another layer of protection. Individual pharmacists may choose not to offer for sale, or refuse requests for certain medicines where they consider the risk of harm outweighs the potential benefits. In the case of theophylline or nitrate preparations, which carry P status in the UK, very few are sold over the counter, thus assuming a pseudo-POM status by convention rather than legislation.

Easy access to medicines for treating minor conditions is recognised as an important part of helping the public to care for their own health, although increasing access also increases the risk of harm. In response to specific concerns of possible harm to the population or individuals, quantity restrictions have been placed on over the counter sales of a number of medicines in the UK, including paracetamol, aspirin, opiate-containing compounds and pseudoephedrine. Paracetamol and aspirin were restricted owing to concern over accidental and deliberate overdose resulting from excessive quantities in the home, while for opiates, the concern relates to the dependency potential arising from long term use. In the case of pseudoephedrine, the risk of harm arises from the ease in which it can be turned into the stimulant metamphetamine, which has caused significant problems in countries such as Australia and the USA (Box 12.1).

Advertising of medicines

In recent years, changes to legislation have led to medicines once again being treated more as normal items of commerce. In the UK, restrictions on advertising for over-the-counter medicines have been lifted and discounts on medicines are now permitted. This could be regarded as a retrograde step in terms of health protection as advertisements sometimes give insufficient information for patients to make informed choices on safe use. Discount offers for medicines could also encourage inappropriate purchases and stockpiling of excessive quantities. In other countries such as the USA, all medicines, including POMs, can be advertised directly to patients. Although this may be beneficial in terms of raising the profile of treatments for certain diseases and increasing awareness, it also carries risks

Box 12.1 *Case study of restriction to pack sizes for pseudoephedrine*

From the early part of the century, illicit production and use of the psychoactive stimulant metamfetamine was recognised as an issue. Illicit production and supply was a significant problem in many countries, particularly Australia and the USA, where supplies of other stimulants on illicit markets were limited. Metamfetamine can be easily produced, without specialist equipment, from household chemicals and pseudoephedrine – a common constituent of many over-the-counter decongestant medicines. Evidence in some countries suggested that criminal gangs were purchasing large quantities of these medicines from pharmacies and using them to produce metamfetamine. As a result, various successful restrictions have been placed on the sale of pseudoephedrine. In the UK, pack size limitations were imposed; in Australia and the USA, records are kept regarding purchasers of pseudoephedrine-containing products. The approach of regulating supplies, rather than simply switching the product's status to POM, is an example of the balancing act between supporting access to medicines needed for treatment of disease and restricting access to prevent harms.

of patients inappropriately requesting medicines from prescribers. Some of the marketing techniques employed can make it difficult for prescribers to promote appropriate use of these medicines through increased pressure to prescribe. There have been calls for such advertising to be permitted in the UK for POMs, but currently this remains very tightly controlled and no promotion to patients is permitted. In all circumstances, health professionals and in particular pharmacists should facilitate the safe and effective use of medicines through educating the public and limiting access to medicines where there is an unacceptable risk of harm to the individual or the public.

Medicines with potential for misuse

The Misuse of Drugs Act consolidated existing legislation relating to drugs with potential for misuse. Replacing the Dangerous Drugs Act, the Misuse of Drugs Act introduced the concept of irresponsible prescribing, tightened security controls and established the Advisory Council on the Misuse of Drugs (ACMD). This panel of experts provides advice to government on scientific evidence relating to harms associated with misuse to support policy decisions regarding managing the risks of these drugs. Drugs listed in the Act, known as controlled drugs, have an identified potential for misuse that warrants control for protection of harm. The purpose of the Act is to prevent the misuse of drugs, while allowing their appropriate medical use. To this end, the Act places controls on the storage, possession, manufacture and supply of a range of medicines and other substances, with the strictest controls being placed on those substances with no accepted medical use and greatest potential for harm. It is under this act that persons importing, supply or using drugs such as heroin, cocaine and cannabis are prosecuted, with the intention to protect both the wider population and individuals through deterrent.

Although controls on supply can reasonably be justified as protecting health, criminalisation of possession for personal use is less clear. In 2004, in response to calls from both professionals working with cannabis users and the police, the UK government, following the advice of the ACMD, reduced penalties for possession and supply of cannabis by reclassification to Class C (reducing penalties to a maximum two years and effectively decriminalising use). However, in 2008, the drug was returned to Class B status (with penalties of up to five years imprisonment for possession and 14 years for supply), against the ACMD's continued advice. This was in response to concerns that decriminalisation had led to wider use and the apparent increased availability and use of stronger types of cannabis, which carried greater risks of harm.

The debate regarding approaches to regulating access to substances of misuse continues in many countries, although most have some restrictions and many are similar to the UK. However, there is considerable variation, with some having more rigorous controls on a wider range of medicines, and others having little control over possession of substances commonly cited as most dangerous – for example, in Portugal, possession of heroin or cocaine results in referral into treatment rather than criminal proceedings. There is evidence that restricting access to substances of abuse merely creates markets for newer substances, as control mechanisms attempt to keep up with illicit markets. One example of this from the UK is a mixture of herbs laced with a series of synthetic cannabinoid receptor agonists, known as 'spice', which was sold as a legal alternative to cannabis. The synthetic agents have higher potency than the main active constituent of cannabis, tetrahydrocannabinol, and have been associated with psychological issues in users, although owing to its relatively recent emergence, its longer term effects are unclear. In December 2009, following ACMD guidance, 'spice' was classified as class B together with all other synthetic cannabinoids. The impact of this reclassification is not yet known, but it is quite likely that yet another 'alternative' will become available to fill the void in the 'legal highs' market.

Looking to the future, health protection in relation to medicines may become even more complex and the ethics clouded with the development and refinement of more drugs that enhance the body's physiological or psychological functioning. Substances such as methyphenidate, sildenafil, androgenic anabolic steroids and human growth hormone are increasingly being used for non-therapeutic reasons by people in many countries. Although this activity is illegal in many of these countries, controls are not enforced to the same degree as with opiate or cocaine use and there is a strong lobby for some of these medicines to be made even more widely available. The difficulty in allowing this arises from the principle of protecting against dangers to health. Although therapeutic use of a medicine is necessary and can be balanced against the potential for harm arising from the medicine, recreational or lifestyle enhancement use of medicines carries no such necessity. The question of how to minimise harm posed by misuse of these and other drugs is explored further in the next section.

Substance use

Approaches to substance use are variable in different countries, ranging from almost complete freedom of access through to severe penalties (including death) for possession and supply. From a public health perspective, criminalisation of substance use has made it difficult to measure and respond to public health needs of substance users owing to the underground nature of the markets and users themselves. The evidence for legal controls on production, supply or use of substances is increasingly coming under scrutiny and is often found lacking. An example is given in Box 12.2.

Box 12.2 *Case study of a policy seeking to prevent substance use through random testing of the general public*

The former USSR state of Georgia introduced a random mandatory drugs testing policy in 2006, with severe fines and confiscation of assets for positive tests. The funds raised by this were not channelled towards drug treatment services or other harm reduction measures, as might have been expected, and the provision of such services was far outstripped by demand. Despite high numbers of positive tests, with some individuals being tested and fined multiple times to the point of bankruptcy, this policy had little effect in preventing the growth of drug use in the country and only served to increase the harms to public health caused by drug use.[1] In 2008, there were signs that the Georgian parliament had realised the policy's ineffectiveness and, partly owing to a desire to join the EU, some proposed it be reviewed.

Indeed, even where the death penalty for trafficking remains in place, there is little evidence that this has any effect on activities. In recent years, there have been widespread calls from all quarters, including law enforcement officers and health professionals, for review of policies to a more evidence-based approach.

Harms associated with substance use

Harm from substance use can include issues such as:

- infected injection sites
- psychological disorders – either directly caused or precipitated in susceptible individuals
- poor overall health – especially dental or nutritional health
- violence associated with the context of use
- systemic infections from contaminated substances or paraphernalia
- overdose
- physiological changes owing to the presence of the drug and physiological damage.

Use of substances such as alcohol and tobacco is well embedded in many cultures throughout the world, while other substances such as opium (the source of morphine) or coca (the source of cocaine) are widely accepted in others. Khat (qat) use is common in countries such as Ethiopia, Kenya and the Yemen, where it is chewed for improved alertness and concentration and its use was noted in pockets of Somali immigrants in the UK in 2005. Despite containing the controlled substances cathinone and cathine, khat is not currently regulated under the Misuse of Drugs Act and its use continues, causing concern in some quarters regarding its deleterious effects on young people.[2]

Controls on the non-therapeutic use of many substances, designed to reduce harm, can often have the unintended effect of introducing new harms through driving use 'underground' into a criminal setting. Most substances available illegally are produced in clandestine facilities, with no quality control mechanisms and where maximising profit is the main driver. In addition, as the substances pass through the supply chain, they are often diluted and adulterated through 'cutting' – a process of dilution with a filler substance, ranging from lactose to plaster or brick dust.

For entirely or partially synthetic drugs, chemical manipulation is often done by inexperienced or poorly qualified people, using improvised equipment. This can result in subtly different chemicals being produced, plus intermediates, sometimes with substantially altered pharmacological action. An example is given in Box 12.3. Consequently, use of illicitly sourced substances poses a greatly increased risk of harm arising from contaminants and overdose owing to the dubious quality and often unknown potency.

Box 12.3 *Case studies of the risks posed by substances produced in clandestine laboratories for illicit markets*

In California in the 1980s, attempts to manufacture the pethidine analogue MPPP in home laboratories resulted in a mixture of MPPP and MPTP. MPTP selectively and irreversibly destroyed the substantia nigra (the brain centre that degrades in Parkinson's disease) in users purchasing and injecting the substance mixture – sold as synthetic pethidine – who developed severe extrapyramidal syndromes shortly after injection.[3] This case was mirrored in eastern Europe and Russia around 2003 to 2006, where methcathinone was being illicitly produced through oxidation of medicines containing ephedrine and pseudoephedrine with potassium permanganate. The resulting chemical mixture contained significant quantities of manganese, which led to development of extrapyramidal syndromes in injecting users.

In addition to the quality of the substances themselves, where injected, further risks arise from the syringes and needles used and the paraphernalia associated with preparation and administration. In a clinical setting, injections are prepared in sterile environments using new, sterilised needles, syringes and filters, pure sterile vehicles (usually water) and solubilising agents. For illicit users, heroin preparation will not usually take place in a sterile environment, or where sterile equipment would readily be available. The drug is usually heated on a spoon with a weak acid to improve solubility. Historically, the weak acid used was food grade (non-sterile) citric or ascorbic acid obtained from pharmacies and supermarkets intended for preparation of jams, or as vitamin tablets. When not available, often because misuse was suspected, vinegar or lemon juice has reportedly been substituted, which carried a risk of blindness from systemic *Candida* infections.

Owing to the presence of insoluble contaminants, an improvised filter is used when drawing the prepared drug into the syringe – often this is a cigarette filter pushed on to the end of the needle. If needles and syringes are not easily available, users commonly retain them for future use and share them with other users. Sharing significantly increases the risks of bacterial infection and transmission of blood borne viruses (such as hepatitis C and HIV). Indeed, data from 2007 show that 90% of people infected with hepatitis C in England, Wales and Northern Ireland were infected through injecting drug use.

Since diamorphine has a short half-life, heroin users need to inject four times each day to minimise withdrawal effects. Given heroin's high cost and the need for regular injections, most users reach a point where most of their day is occupied obtaining supplies or funds to purchase supplies (often through criminal activity). This leads to a very chaotic lifestyle, making it difficult to maintain a job and often alienating the user from social networks beyond their fellow users.

Other products with misuse potential

Over recent decades, there has been a substantial increase in use of substances to alter appearance or performance, known collectively known as performance and image enhancing drugs (PIEDs). Historically this was restricted to drugs and food supplements to enhance muscle growth among professional athletes and bodybuilders, but the use of these substances is growing rapidly among more casual users, seeking a media-led 'perfect' body or attempting to gain an edge in academic pursuits.

Substances used to alter physical appearance include androgenic anabolic steroids, growth hormone and a range of substances marketed as food supplements, intended to supply protein for muscle growth or increase metabolic rate through training to reduce fat. Additionally, a range of other drugs are used to further enhance the image (e.g. diuretics to enhance muscle definition) or counter adverse reactions (e.g. tamoxifen to counter gynaecomastia). The use of these substances carries many risks, including: adverse reactions to substances, complex interactions when multiple substances are used together, risks from injecting, and counterfeit or contaminated products in the supply chain.

Other drugs used illicitly to alter physical appearance are the synthetic melanocortin analogues afamelanotide (melanotan I) and melanotan II.[4] These unlicensed drugs act on melanocytes to stimulate production of melanin and lead to a deep tan following a course of injections. These drugs (in common with many PIEDs) have become widely available through the internet, where anonymity allows sellers and purchasers to operate with little risk of prosecution. Owing to the nature of the supply chain, the products purchased are again of dubious quality or potency. Since these drugs have not completed clinical trials, little safety data are available, although their use has been linked to cases of rapid mole alteration including dysplastic nevus – a form of mole closely associated with melanoma.[5] In addition to the obvious risks of using untested medicines bought through illicit supply chains, there is a much more worrying issue in the administration of injections by largely naive individuals. Anecdotal reports from drugs agency workers include examples of up to six friends sharing a single needle, syringe and multi-use injection vial for daily injections over a two-week period. Such behaviour carries a substantial risk of transmission of blood-borne viruses and also nerve or other cellular damage through use of blunt needles, with a high likelihood of colonisation by bacterial or fungal species.

Recent pharmaceutical developments and wider clinical use has also led to an increasing trend towards the non-therapeutic use of 'smart' drugs, such as modafinil and methylphenidate. These are used therapeutically in conditions such as narcolepsy or attention deficit disorders, but are increasingly used with the intention of enhancing concentration. Additionally, cognitive enhancing products being developed for therapeutic use in dementia and other cognitive disorders are increasingly becoming available on illicit markets and used to enhance cognitive function in otherwise healthy individuals.

In addition to the issues outlined above, as more drugs are developed for therapeutic uses and more imaginative applications made to existing products, the use of drugs to alter physical and mental performance or image is likely to continue to rise and evolve, introducing many complex new problems.

Reducing harms associated with substance use

Despite the legal controls placed on supply and use of these medicines, they continue to be used and generate public health issues. For this reason, the concept of harm reduction, or harm minimisation, has become widely accepted among the health professions and, in some countries, policy makers. Harm reduction encompasses interventions and activities intended to minimise the harms associated with the non-therapeutic use of substances. The ethos of harm reduction is not to prevent use, but to minimise the risks through education and intervention, reducing the extent of use and the risks associated with remaining use. A number of pharmacy-related activities are associated with harm reduction in most sectors of practice.

In the context of community pharmacy, harm reduction often relates to services associated with use of opiates and injectable substances such as stimulants and some PIEDs. Community pharmacies have been involved in providing needle and syringe programmes (NSPs) in some countries for many years (see Chapter 5) and represent approximately four in five NSP outlets in England and Scotland.

NSPs are concerned with reducing harms associated with injection of substances – primarily opiates, stimulants and steroids – and provide disposable, sterile needles and syringes with sharps bins for safe disposal. In addition, many NSPs provide sterile paraphernalia used in the preparation and administration of opiates, including: citric or ascorbic acid (to acidify base heroin for improved solubility), single use 'cookers' (small metal dishes with a handle) for heating the heroin mix, filters for minimising the particulates in the injection and alcohol swabs for cleaning the injection site prior to administration. Information leaflets on subjects such as safe injection techniques are also provided in some services.

The other key harm reduction service provided through UK community pharmacies is substitution therapy, which is also provided in many countries (see Chapter 5). This involves substituting illicit opiates with a stable, free supply to reduce injection, minimise criminal activity (associated with obtaining funds for purchase of illicit supplies) and enabling the individual to regain control of their life. Historically, detoxification was seen as the main aim of substitution therapy, but maintenance is now seen as a useful intervention in its own right. Given the harm reduction aim of substitution, there is little value in reducing the dose of the substitute more rapidly than the user is able to cope with, since this will likely lead to a return to injecting and the associated risks. Additionally, rapid detoxification limits the possible benefits that might be seen in building a stable life, including undertaking training or re-entering work, as well as re-establishing familial and other social relationships. Substitution is usually in the form of oral methadone, primarily as a mixture or solution, but also in tablet form for those who cannot tolerate the liquid. Sometimes it may be difficult to stabilise the patient on oral methadone and injectable methadone may be used, particularly where there is psychological dependency associated with the injection process. More recently, sublingual buprenorphine has also been used in substitution therapy. This has the advantage of a long half-life, resulting in a slower onset of withdrawal effects if doses are delayed or missed and can be useful in patients whose life remains chaotic. In rare cases, it may prove necessary to use pharmaceutical diamorphine as the substitute drug, but this requires specific licensing of the prescriber in the UK and is used infrequently. Some studies have shown it to be potentially beneficial in those who are difficult to treat, but its use is associated with increased risk of adverse effects and is likely to remain limited.

Many community pharmacies also observe the consumption of the substitute drug, particularly when a user is first initiated. This has two key benefits from a harm reduction perspective: it provides a regular, structured contact between a user and a health professional and it ensures that the correct dose is being taken regularly. The latter helps to avoid risks of overdose and preventing diversion of substitute therapies into illicit markets.

There is often confusion among service providers when a patient receiving substitution therapy is also obtaining needles from an NSP. It is important to remember that the aim of harm reduction is to reduce harm to as low a level as possible and, at least initially, it may only be possible to reduce use of illicit opiates to once or twice per week, rather than reaching a complete substitution state. Clearly this significantly reduces the risk compared with normal use of up to 30 injections per week, therefore achieves harm reduction. This not only protects the individual's health, but also the wider population through lower population infection rates of blood-borne viruses and reduced crime.

The easy accessibility of the pharmacist, including late opening hours and convenient location are often cited as benefits of pharmacy-based NSPs. Alongside the rapport that can be built between pharmacy staff and users of pharmacy services through regular contact, this provides many opportunities for ad hoc interventions. Therefore, community pharmacies are well placed to provide further support to help protect against the harms associated with substance use. Other services might include:

- supporting users in maintaining their general health
- supporting stopping smoking or moderating alcohol intake
- ensuring good nutrition and dental care
- inspection of injection sites and providing advice on wound care
- screening for sexually transmitted and other infectious diseases
- vaccinations.

Initially pioneered by Australia, supervised injecting facilities have now been introduced by many European countries. These centres are usually manned by trained healthcare staff and allow injection of drugs such as heroin – sometimes supplied by the centre – in a clean environment, using appropriate and sterile equipment. Injections are still administered by the drug users themselves, although some also provide advice on injection technique and support in minimising the harms associated with injection. Additionally, resuscitation equipment and drugs such as naloxone are available and staff can respond immediately to an overdose, substantially reducing the risk of death.

In countries where they are implemented, these facilities are part of a wider range of services and help to promote treatment services such as methadone maintenance and psychosocial support, further helping to reduce harms. A study in Sydney, Australia during 2001/2 estimated that the facility helped to save four lives per annum and prevented a rise in hepatitis B and C infection rates among its users, while infections rates rose elsewhere in the country.[6] Where centres have engaged with the community, there is evidence that they improve the local area for all residents, with less street-based injection and fewer discarded needles. In addition, the incidence of ambulance callouts associated with illicit opiate overdose is significantly reduced in the vicinity of injecting facilities, thereby reducing the impact of illicit opiate use on other emergency treatment.

Communicable diseases

A communicable disease is one where the agent causing the disease can spread from individual to individual through one of a range of transmission routes. Transmission routes include:

- direct contact with infected body fluids of an infected individual

- contact with an object that has been contaminated by an infected individual
- vectors such as mosquitoes, flies and other insects.

The spread of communicable diseases is one of the most significant health threats to humans throughout the world, including both developing and developed countries (see Chapter 5), in part, as these diseases are often difficult to treat once contracted. However, in many countries, the risks posed by communicable diseases have been substantially reduced through health protection measures that seek to minimise transmission and contain outbreaks where possible. Owing to the rapidly changing nature of infectious diseases and the development of resistance, it is also important to control the treatment mechanisms to minimise the risks of resistance developing, particularly for bacterial infections.

Notification of certain diseases is one strategic mechanism designed to provide intelligence on disease spread. This can then be controlled, through containment, use of chemical prophylaxis agents, and through hygiene measures. Educating health professionals and the general public on the importance of good hygiene is also an important mechanism to minimise disease spread, particularly in the case of infections transmitted through non-contact mechanisms (e.g. influenza). Periodically, where specific threats exist – e.g. influenza in 2009 – information is issued, in this case, advising people to dispose of used tissues and regularly wash hands when infected or in contact with infected individuals.

Pharmacists have a number of important roles in supporting health protection measures to combat communicable diseases; these include recognition and referral of infected individuals, education and advice on minimising risk of transmission (including hygiene measures) and providing vaccinations for difficult to reach groups.

Vaccination

Vaccinations are one of the most useful mechanisms in protecting a population from the risks associated with communicable diseases. Indeed, as a result of the development of the smallpox vaccine, the World Health Organization officially reported in 1980 that smallpox had been completely eradicated worldwide.

In most developed countries, a standard vaccination programme for a range of diseases begins at childhood and continues throughout adolescence. The primary intention of these vaccination programmes is to protect individuals against the harms associated with contracting the disease itself. However, it also has a secondary benefit associated with population immunity. Population (or herd) immunity relates to the situation whereby a disease that normally passes from person to person within a population cannot spread so easily where most of the population are immune to the disease. This is because immune individuals do not act as a point of infection, so cannot pass the disease on to others. Such population immunity not only protects the vaccinated individuals through their own immunity but also protects people who cannot be vaccinated owing to age or other complications such as immunodeficiency. The threshold at which population immunity is reached is difficult to model and differs between diseases, although figures ranging from 55 to 95% have been proposed for measles.[7]

In the UK, the immunisation programme has successfully led to once common conditions being rare, with fewer individuals contracting the disease and fewer deaths as a result. This is, as with all immunisation programmes, related to the population as well as individual immunity. All health professionals, including pharmacists, have a role in appropriately promoting vaccination and providing a consistent message in line with current practice to ensure population immunity thresholds are maintained. One example where this was made clear was seen in the UK in the late 1990s involving an academic paper, which has since been retracted, that incorrectly linked autism with the measles, mumps and rubella vaccine leading to substantial decline in parents consenting to their children receiving it. Over the following decade, as the population and individual immunity fell, cases of measles rose to ten times previous levels.

Vaccination programmes are routinely reviewed and updated in light of current threats to the population. This may be an ongoing threat or a specific emergency situation where a new strain of infection has begun spreading. One example of this is the human papillomavirus (HPV). HPV is implicated in over 70% of cases of cervical cancer, which, in the UK, is the twelfth most common cancer affecting women and causes approximately 1000 deaths each year.[8] In 2008, a vaccine for HPV was added to the standard regimen for 12–13-year-old girls in the UK with the intention that vaccinated women will be protected from infection and consequently developing cervical cancer. In addition, over time, the presence of HPV will decline, substantially reducing the risks of cervical cancer in all women, including those who have not received the vaccine. HPV vaccinations have already been shown to reduce the incidence of cervical cell abnormalities and even protect against genital warts. Taking population immunity principles to an extreme, some have even suggested that HPV vaccination be extended to men, despite the fact that infection poses no risk to them.

Seasonal influenza is routinely seen in many countries and affects tens of thousands of people each year. Most people will have some degree of immunity to many of the strains and will either not contract the illness or have a mild to moderate infection. However, the elderly and those with weakened immune systems or underlying conditions are at risk of serious complications from influenza and in some cases, this can lead to death. For this reason, authorities in many countries identify the strain(s) most likely to be prevalent each winter and a vaccination is offered to vulnerable groups for these strains. Additionally, increasing numbers of community pharmacies in the UK offer vaccination privately for people not eligible for the free NHS service. The influenza virus, in common with most viruses, undergoes two types of evolutionary change that continually challenge individuals' immune systems. These are known as antigenic drift and antigenic shift. In the case of drift, the virus undergoes minor mutations during reproduction, which results in subtle changes to the virus, allowing it to infect previously immune individuals. Seasonal influenza undergoes this process and it is through prediction of which shifts will be most prevalent that appropriate vaccines are developed. In the case of shift, an influenza virus that does not presently infect humans exchanges genes with one that does. This leads to development of a new strain of virus, for which there is very little immunity in the general population.

In the case of antigenic shift, major epidemics and even pandemics can develop – for example, the influenza pandemic of 1918–19, which resulted from a shift, with avian (bird) influenza beginning to infect humans and causing 40–50 million deaths worldwide. Three further pandemics have been recorded, one in 1957, one in 1968 and one in 2009. In each case, a new influenza strain has developed the ability to infect humans and there is little underlying immunity, particularly among children and younger adults who have been exposed to fewer strains during their lifetime. Where major outbreaks of communicable diseases arise, or are anticipated, it is essential that strategic emergency planning is implemented to ensure that appropriate containment measures are ensured and that safe and effective treatments can be provided where needed (Box 12.4). Further information on emergency planning is given in Chapter 1.

Antimicrobial resistance

Since the development of penicillin in the mid-20th century, the prognosis for an individual with a bacterial infection has substantially improved. There are now many different antibiotic agents, acting on a range of different components in the bacterial cell and active against a range of bacteria types. However, owing to the rapid rate of replication and mutation of bacterial cells, resistance has developed to many antibiotics, resulting in some now being only of limited use. It has thus become necessary to use more toxic agents in an attempt to treat infections that have been colonised by multi-drug resistant strains of bacteria such as *Staphylococcus aureus*.

Box 12.4 *Case study of the UK response to the swine flu pandemic*

When the highly virulent H1N1 strain of influenza was first noted in Mexico, health protection agencies worldwide began examining the risks to their nation's population. In the UK, government worked to develop an appropriate response to the outbreak. Given the significant likelihood of transmission, this strain was initially very concerning. In response to the risk, stockpiles of antiviral medication that had already partially accrued owing to previous threats of pandemic influenza were increased and advanced orders for vaccines were placed with pharmaceutical companies who immediately began development. Initially, the policy sought to contain infections and antivirals were issued to close contacts of infected individuals. However, once infection became more widespread, this policy was changed to treating only infected individuals with antivirals, but minimising spread though requiring a representative to collect medication. Community pharmacies were used by many primary care trusts as collection points and in England a telephone triage system was created, which allowed representatives of infected individuals to access antivirals without needing a prescription. Towards the end of 2009, once clinical trials of the vaccine had been completed, all vulnerable groups and frontline healthcare workers were offered the vaccine. Although the H1N1 strain generally caused only mild symptoms in infected patients, there was a greater risk in those with underlying medical conditions and a substantial risk to continuity of healthcare services if large numbers of healthcare staff were absent from work owing to sickness.

Resistance is a worrying development in the treatment of bacterial infections as specific mechanisms of resistance can spread from one bacterium to another, leading to effective redundancy of drugs in some cases. Resistance develops as a result of a number of scenarios, but the most common are excessive use – in patients that are gaining minimal clinical benefit – and sub therapeutic doses or short treatment lengths. In the latter scenario, if 95% of a bacterial colony has been killed, it is likely that the remaining 5% will contain a proportionately high degree of resistance. Continued treatment (and the host's own immune system) would likely eradicate the remaining bacteria. However, if treatment is stopped prematurely, the bacteria will grow back with a greater level of resistance than before the course began. Subsequent attempts to treat this infection will likely be less successful unless a different antibiotic is used. The same is true where a subtherapeutic dose is used, selectively killing those bacteria without resistance, leaving a greater proportion of resistant strains to flourish when the treatment ceases. Clearly each occasion an antibiotic is used will lead to selective death of non-resistant strains and leave only the resistant ones alive. In normal circumstances, this greatly reduced number will be tackled by the host's own immune system. However, on occasions, the bacteria may transfer to another host, carrying the resistance capacity with it. Through plasmid exchange, this resistance may spread through a number of other bacterial strains and these spread across more hosts, gaining other resistance mechanisms along the way. Thus, the more a given antibiotic is used, the more resistance to it will exist in the bacterial population and the greater the likelihood that treatment with that drug will be ineffective. Bacterial strains such as vancomycin-resistant enterococci or methicillin-resistant *Staphylococcus aureus* (MRSA) are popularly known as 'superbugs' as they have developed substantial resistance and are particularly difficult to treat, giving rise to serious complications in patients with underlying medical conditions.

As illustrated above, widespread inappropriate use of antibiotics can render individual drugs ineffective and community pharmacists in many countries have a public health role in promoting the appropriate use of antibiotic preparations. In particular, providing advice on appropriate treatment of viral infections such as common colds or influenza can substantially reduce antibiotic use. In addition, many countries have limited the availability of antibiotics to protect the wider community by minimising the potential for resistance. In the UK, this restriction has historically been through limiting all antibiotics to POM status, but recently a few drugs have been reclassified to P medicine status, including: chloramphenicol products for eye infections; azithromycin for chlamydial infections and nitrofurantoin for urinary tract infections. This shift has substantially altered the role of community pharmacists in terms of managing antibiotic use and the deregulation was resisted because of concerns about the risks of resistance. Community pharmacists now have a duty to assess presenting conditions to make sound judgements about the necessity for supplying a P medicine. Without such controls, free availability would likely render these substantially less effective owing to widespread unnecessary use. In the UK community pharmacists' practices are being closely monitored and it is likely that the impacts of the deregulation of these agents will influence further deregulation of antibiotic preparations in future.

In restricting access, it is also necessary to control which agents are used in which contexts – effectively restricting access to health professionals as well – such that treatment choices are maximised. To this end, antibiotic formularies are widely implemented in secondary and primary care trusts.

These formularies take account of local resistance patterns and the relative risks of each antibiotic therapy, making recommendations on which agency should be used for which infections. In addition to this, local policies also usually require practitioners to swab infections where possible and have specific resistance identified such that the most effective treatment for the individual can be used – and consequently, gain maximum benefit with minimal risk of resistance.

References

1. Otiashvili D, Sárosi P, Somogyi GL. *Briefing Paper 15. Drug Control in Georgia: Drug testing and the reduction of drug use?* Beckley, Oxon: Beckley Foundation, 2008. http://www.beckleyfoundation.org/pdf/BriefingPaper_15.pdf
2. Advisory Council on the Misuse of Drugs. *Khat (Qat): Assessment of risk to the individual and communities in the UK.* London: Home Office, 2005. http://drugs.homeoffice.gov.uk/publication-search/acmd/khat-report-2005/
3. Williams A. MPTP parkinsonism. *BMJ* 1984; 289(6456): 1401.
4. Evans-Brown M, Dawson RT, Chandler M *et al.* Use of melanotan I and II in the general population. *BMJ* 2009; 338: 566.
5. Langan EA, Ramlogan D, Jamieson LA *et al.* Change in moles linked to use of unlicensed 'sun tan jab'. *BMJ* 2009; 338: b277.
6. Allison MS, Ingrid van B, Janaki A *et al.* The impact of a supervised injecting facility on ambulance call-outs in Sydney, Australia. *Addiction* 2010; 105(4): 676–683. doi:10.1111/j.1360-0443.2009.02837.x.
7. May T, Silverman R. 'Clustering of exemptions' as a collective action threat to herd immunity. *Vaccine* 2003; 21(11–12): 1048–1051.
8. Munoz N, Kjaer SK, Sigurdsson K *et al.* Impact of human papillomavirus (HPV)-6/11/16/18 vaccine on all HPV-associated genital diseases in young women. *J Natl Cancer Inst* 2010; 102 (5):325–339. doi:10.1093/jnci/djp534.

Suggested reading

Appleby GE, Wingfield J. *Dale and Appelbe's Pharmacy Law and Ethics,* 9th edn. London: Pharmaceutical Press, 2009.

Department of Health, the Scottish Government, Welsh Assembly Government, Northern Ireland Executive. *Drug Misuse and Dependence: UK guidelines on clinical management.* London: Department of Health (England), the Scottish Government, Welsh Assembly Government and Northern Ireland Executive, 2007.

Gossop M. Classification of illegal and harmful drugs. *BMJ* 2006; 333(7562): 272–273.

Health Protection Agency Centre for Infections, Health Protection Scotland, National Public Health Service for Wales, Communicable Disease Surveillance Centre Northern Ireland, Centre for Research on Drugs & Health Behaviour, London School of Hygiene and Tropical Medicine. *Shooting Up: Infections among injecting drug users in the United Kingdom 2007. An update: October 2008.* London: Health Protection Agency, 2008.

Lawrie T, Matheson C, Bond CM *et al.* Pharmacy customers' views and experiences of using pharmacies which provide drug misuse services. *Drug Alcohol Rev* 2004 Jun; 23(2): 195–202.

National Institute for Health and Clinical Excellence. *Needle and Syringe Programmes: Providing people who inject drugs with injecting equipment.* London: NICE, 2009.

Salisbury D, Ramsay M, Noakes K, editors. *Immunisation against Infectious Disease*, 3rd edn. London: TSO, 2006.

Strang J, Fortson R. Supervised fixing rooms, supervised injectable maintenance clinics: understanding the difference. *BMJ* 2004; 328(7431): 102–103.

Taheri L. Testing for hepatitis in pharmacies. *Pharm J* 2010; 284: 51.

Walker M. *Best Practice Guidance for Commissioners and Providers of Pharmaceutical Services to Drug Users*. London: National Treatment Agency, 2006.

Wills S. *Drugs of Abuse*, 2nd edn. London: Pharmaceutical Press, 2005.

Wright NMJ, Tompkins CNE. Supervised injecting centres. *British Medical Journal* 2004; 328: 100–102.

13

Preventing disease: screening in the pharmacy

Ines Krass and Carol Armour

Screening is the systematic application of a test process to people who have not previously sought medical attention for a disorder, to identify individuals at sufficient risk of the disorder to warrant further investigation.[1] It is not a service in itself, but is a component of a wider strategy that may include diagnosis, and always includes a plan of action for health promotion and the prevention or control of the disease.[2] The term *screening* implies the use of laboratory or point of care tests, but may involve the use of risk assessment questionnaires, physical examination, observation alone or may combine methods.

Although when effectively implemented, screening can save lives or improve quality of life through early diagnosis of serious conditions, its application requires careful assessment of risks and benefits. For example, screening can reduce the risk of developing a condition or its complications but cannot guarantee total protection. Screening is also subject to error and any screening programme will result in a proportion of false positive results (wrongly reported as having the condition) and false negative results (wrongly reported as not having the condition). False positive results in cancer screening have produced high levels of anxiety that do not resolve immediately when subsequent testing shows no signs of the disease.[1]

There is a need to establish the extent to which screening can prevent disability and premature death and balance this against the financial and human costs of anxiety, discomfort, adverse effects, follow-up investigations and unnecessary treatments. As a general principle therefore, screening should only target diseases or disorders known to cause significant suffering, disability or death if detected at a later stage.

Principles of screening

There are three broad approaches to screening:

- population based

- selective
- opportunistic case detection.

Population-based approaches attempt to screen everybody, selective screening targets groups at high risk and opportunistic case detection involves providing a screening test to individuals during routine encounters with the healthcare system.[3]

According to the World Health Organization, population-based screening in asymptomatic populations is only appropriate if all of the following conditions are met[1]:

- The disease is a significant health problem.
- The natural history of the disease is understood.
- There is an identifiable preclinical stage of the disease.
- Tests are reliable.
- The benefits of treatment after early detection are better than those obtained if treatment is delayed.
- The process is cost-effective.
- The screening will be a systematic ongoing process.

Assessing the effectiveness of screening

The validity of a screening test is determined in terms of its sensitivity and specificity, defined in Tables 13.1a and 13.1b. High sensitivity indicates that a test is successful in detecting people affected by the disease. Specificity does the reverse by producing evidence that a test is identifying people who do not have the disease (false positives). Although it is desirable to have a test that is both highly sensitive and highly specific, this is usually not possible. In choosing a cut-off point a trade-off needs to be made between sensitivity and specificity, as increasing one reduces the other.[1]

The predictive value of a test is determined not only by its sensitivity and specificity, but also by the prevalence of the disorder in the screened population. Thus, a highly sensitive and specific test will have a high positive predictive value in a population with a high prevalence of the disorder. This is part of the rationale for promoting selective or targeted screening. When the prevalence is low, the predictive value will be considerably lower, so a high specificity drives a high value. To avoid false positives (throughout the range of prevalence), it may be necessary to increase specificity at the expense of sensitivity.[1]

Another measure of the accuracy of a screening test is given by the area under a receiver operating characteristic (ROC) curve. This is a plot of the true positive rate against the false positive rate for the different possible cut-points of a diagnostic test. Values range from 0 to 1. An area of 1 represents a perfect test; an area of 0.5 represents a worthless test (Figure 13.1).

Table 13.1a Classification of screening test results

Test result	Affected	Unaffected
Positive	*a*	*b*
Negative	*c*	*d*

Table 13.1b Definitions

Term	Definition	Formula
Sensitivity or detection rate (DR)	Proportion of affected individuals with positive results	$a/a + c$
Specificity	Proportion of unaffected individuals with negative results	$d/b + d$ or $1 -$ false positive rate
False positive rate	Proportion of unaffected individuals with positive results	$b/b + d$ or $1 -$ specificity
Positive predictive value (PPV)	Probability that an affected individual has the disease	$a/a + b$
Odds of being affected given a positive results (OAPR)	Ratio of the number of affected to unaffected individuals among those with positive results	$a : b$
Adapted from Strong *et al.*[1]		

Evidence for the effectiveness of screening programmes

Much of the evidence for the benefits of screening is indirect, derived from clinical trials where only those people identified as positive through the screening test are randomised to be treated or not. Definitive evidence of

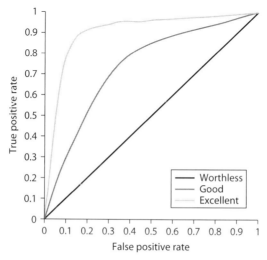

Figure 13.1 Illustration of the value of receiver operating characteristic (ROC) curves using differing cut-off points for positive results. From http://gim.unmc.edu/dxtests/roc2.htm with permission.

effectiveness of screening can only be demonstrated by a randomised controlled trial, where the only difference between intervention and control groups is exposure to the screening test itself.[1]

To date, few robust trials have been conducted to assess the effectiveness of screening programmes in decreasing mortality and morbidity. Studies providing treatments to a screened group but not to a control group are rare because of feasibility and ethical concerns related to denying treatment to a diagnosed patient. Moreover, because the benefits of screening may be small and accrue over a long period, the number of patients needed for such studies are substantial, making the research very costly.

In the UK, a national screening committee advises the government on all aspects of screening policy. Its brief is to use research evidence, pilot programmes and economic evaluations to recommend the adoption of screening programmes that do more good than harm at a reasonable cost.[4] The committee also manages some screening programmes, except those for cancer and those which they have not approved. A list of all current national screening programmes in England is given in Table 13.2. A newly established body in Australia, the Australian Screening Advisory Committee, provides advice on existing national screening programmes, those under consideration and emerging screening issues in relation to cancer.[5]

Many opportunities present for community pharmacists to provide screening tests on an opportunistic basis and to become involved in national screening programmes. Currently there are only two national programmes in the UK in which pharmacists have been identified as having a major role; however, this chapter and Chapter 11 also include other examples. Many of these should be regarded as opportunistic testing, rather than screening. However, such opportunities are part of the advantage that pharmacists have over other health professionals.

Screening for diagnosis of non-communicable diseases

Type 2 diabetes

Background

Type 2 diabetes is the most common non-communicable disease globally and the fourth or fifth leading cause of death in developed countries, arising mainly from cardiovascular disease. Other complications such as neuropathy, nephropathy and retinopathy also contribute to mortality and disabilities. Global prevalence is rising rapidly, but at least 50% of all people with type 2 diabetes are unaware of their condition or that they are at significant risk of developing diabetes.[6] In this so called prediabetic state, where people have either impaired glucose tolerance or impaired fasting glucose, damage to blood vessels and nerves may already be underway.[7]

Table 13.2 Screening programmes operating in England

Screening programme	Target population/purpose	Approved by UK National Screening Committee
Fetal anomaly	Ultrasound for all pregnant women, to assess for physical anomalies and offer Down's syndrome screening	Yes
Infectious diseases in pregnancy	All pregnant women, offered screening for hepatitis B, HIV, rubella susceptibility and syphilis	Yes
Sickle cell and thalassaemia	All pregnant women, to identify sickle cell disease	Yes
Newborn blood spot	All babies at birth, to screen for phenylketonuria, congenital hypothyroidism, sickle cell disease, cystic fibrosis and medium-chain acyl-CoA dehydrogenase deficiency	Yes
Newborn hearing	All babies within two weeks of birth, to identify all children born with moderate to profound permanent bilateral deafness	Yes
Abdominal aortic aneurysm	Men at age 65, to identify and treat or monitor aneurysms	Yes, being gradually introduced
Diabetic retinopathy	Annually, to people with diabetes aged 12 or over, to reduce risk of sight loss	Yes
Breast	Women aged 50 to 70 every three years, to detect and treat breast cancer early	Yes
Cervical	Women aged 25 to 50 every three years, aged 50 to 64 every five years, to detect and treat cervical abnormalities	Yes
Bowel cancer	People between 60 and 70 every two years, to detect and treat bowel cancer	Yes
Prostate cancer	Provide opportunity to men concerned about prostate cancer to have a prostate-specific antigen test	No
Chlamydia	Young people under 25, to identify disease and ensure management	No
Health check	People between 40 and 74, not already diagnosed with heart disease, stroke or diabetes, to reduce risk and ensure disease management	No

During its relatively long asymptomatic phase, it can easily be identified by the presence of post-prandial and/or fasting hyperglycaemia through reliable laboratory blood testing procedures, well before typical symptoms develop. Moreover, it has been shown that earlier diagnosis of type 2 diabetes is associated with better outcomes.[8] More recently, several trials[9,10] have demonstrated the benefits of early interventions (lifestyle or metformin) for patients with impaired glucose tolerance detected through a screening programme, which strengthens the case for screening. Currently, the ADDITION trial (a randomised controlled trial to provide evidence of the long term benefits, harms and costs of implementing a screening and early treatment programme for type 2 diabetes) is under way but will not report for about 5 years.[11]

Whether or not screening is cost-effective depends on the approach used. Population-based approaches are very costly and inefficient because of the relatively low prevalence of diabetes in the community. Both selective screening and opportunistic case detection require fewer resources[1]; however, if conducted in the general community, they may be less effective than hoped because of the failure of people who test positively to seek and obtain appropriate follow up for diagnostic testing and care.[1] Opportunistic case detection may be the best option for type 2 diabetes.[8] Internationally, approaches to screening for type 2 diabetes vary. However, in general the recommendations focus on screening of high risk individuals.[10,11]

Methods of screening for diabetes

Screening tests for type 2 diabetes include risk assessment questionnaires, biochemical tests in the form of blood glucose measurement and combinations of these.

Risk scores based on a combination of risk factors are increasingly being used as the initial step in identifying people who should undergo blood glucose testing. Table 13.3 summarises some examples of available questionnaires and their characteristics. While they vary in the factors used to assess risk, most demonstrate similar levels of sensitivity, specificity and accuracy (receiver operating characteristic values). Factors common to all tools include age, family history of diabetes, elevated blood pressure, BMI more than 25 kg/m^2 and insufficient physical activity.

Most screening protocols recommend a follow-up screening blood test for individuals identified to be at risk, by either a laboratory test using venous plasma glucose or a capillary blood glucose test using a point of care (POC) device. The advantages of POC testing centre on the convenience and accessibility of testing, which may increase participation in screening and adherence to follow-up diagnostics processes.[8] There are concerns about the accuracy of these devices and the lack of equivalence of venous plasma and capillary blood glucose. Recently a change in the Australian guidelines reflects a shift in favour of capillary blood glucose as a permissible alternative to laboratory testing.[12] POC testing is also viewed as acceptable for use in pharmacies in the UK.

Table 13.3 Selected diabetes risk screening tools

Risk scale	Score range: cut point	Factors included	Sensitivity	Specificity	ROC
Danish diabetes risk score	0–60: >31	Age, sex, family history of diabetes, elevated blood pressure, BMI >25 kg/m², insufficient physical activity	76%	72%	0.8
Cambridge risk score (CRS)	0–1: > 0.199	Age, gender, BMI, steroid and antihypertensive medication, family and smoking history	77%	72%	0.8
Finnish diabetes risk score (FINDRISC)	0–26: >11	Age, BMI, waist circumference, physical activity, daily consumption of fruits, berries and vegetables, history of antihypertensive drug treatment, history of blood glucose, family history of diabetes	66% for females; 70% for males	69% for females; 61% for males	0.73 for females; 0.72 for males
The Australian Type 2 diabetes risk assessment tool (AUSDRISK)	0–36: <12	Age, sex, ethnicity, family history of diabetes, hypertension, smoking, fruit and vegetable consumption, history of blood glucose, waist circumference, physical activity	78%	58%	0.75

Adapted from Colagiuri et al.[8]
ROC = receiver operating characteristic.

A three-step process for case detection and diagnosis of individuals at high risk of type 2 diabetes is illustrated in Figure 13.2 derived from Australian guidelines.[8]

Opportunities for pharmacy screening

Community pharmacy provides a logical site for this, with its established, expansive and visible network of easily accessible health professionals. Importantly, community pharmacists can access a broad, apparently healthy, population who rarely come into contact with GPs or nurses. The consumer

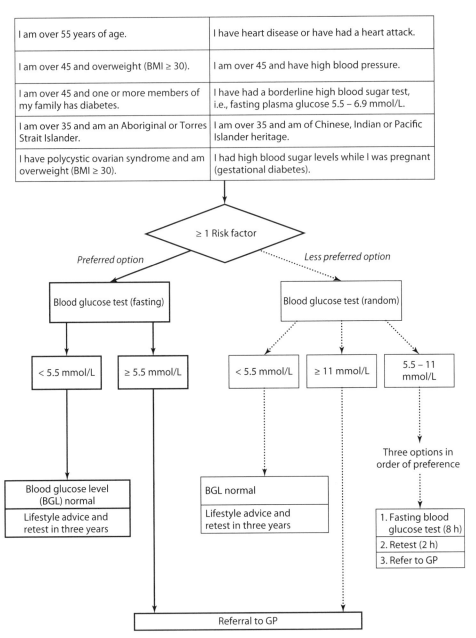

I am over 55 years of age.	I have heart disease or have had a heart attack.
I am over 45 and overweight (BMI ≥ 30).	I am over 45 and have high blood pressure.
I am over 45 and one or more members of my family has diabetes.	I have had a borderline high blood sugar test, i.e., fasting plasma glucose 5.5 – 6.9 mmol/L.
I am over 35 and am an Aboriginal or Torres Strait Islander.	I am over 35 and am of Chinese, Indian or Pacific Islander heritage.
I have polycystic ovarian syndrome and am overweight (BMI ≥ 30).	I had high blood sugar levels while I was pregnant (gestational diabetes).

Figure 13.2   Sequential screening protocol for risk assessment (based on NHMRC guidelines). From reference 16. Reproduced with permission.

may consult a pharmacist without an appointment and often with minimal waiting times. Moreover, pharmacists can use their available information on medicines and health conditions to identify people at possible risk who should be screened, as well as providing education and referral.

Evidence for pharmacy screening

Over the past decade, a number of community pharmacy-based diabetes screening programmes have been trialled and implemented. A national survey of Australian community pharmacies in 2002 reported that approximately 79 000 screening tests for glucose had been conducted in the previous year with 22% of pharmacies conducting at least one test per month.[13] Approaches to screening have varied across settings. Others have focused exclusively on risk assessment (step 1) only, such as a pilot project in Belgian community pharmacies that involved disseminating risk assessment questionnaires to customers who were advised to consult their physician if they had more than one risk factor. This study showed that 20 patients needed to be screened to diagnose one person with diabetes.[14]

In 2004, an screening trial in 28 randomly selected Australian community pharmacies compared the efficacy and cost-effectiveness of screening for risk factors with a tick test (risk assessment) alone to steps 1 and 2 of the sequential screening process outlined in Figure 13.2. A total of 1286 people were screened over three months and the rate of diabetes diagnosis was significantly higher for sequential screening compared with the tick test (1.7% versus 0.2%; p = 0.008). It also resulted in fewer referrals to the GP and a higher uptake of referrals than the tick test, so was the more cost-effective screening method.[12]

A national Swiss self care campaign called 'Stop-diabetes-test now' also used the sequential screening approach in 530 community pharmacies, together with the transtheoretical model (see Chapter 11) to assess motivation to change behaviour and lifestyle counselling by pharmacists. Of the 98 258 persons screened, 6.9% were detected with possible diabetes and 74% received targeted lifestyle advice.[15] An American study focusing on minority populations and the elderly found that sequential screening for both diabetes and cardiovascular disease in 577 community pharmacies resulted in greater uptake of physician referral than screening provided in 331 non-healthcare settings (51% versus 42%).[16]

Collectively these studies support the feasibility of screening for diabetes in community pharmacy and highlight the additional opportunity for the pharmacist to engage in health promotion and prevention counselling.

Cardiovascular disease

Background

Cardiovascular disease is a leading cause of death, morbidity and disability in developed and developing countries and imposes an enormous and escalating clinical, economic and public health burden. Globally, an estimated 17.5

million people died from cardiovascular disease in 2005, representing 30% of all deaths. Of these deaths, almost half were due to heart attacks and a third caused by stroke.[17] While the manifestations of cardiovascular disease usually occur only in middle age and thereafter, the underlying pathological process, namely atherosclerosis, commences early in life and progresses slowly such that there is a long asymptomatic period. A number of significant modifiable risk factors influence disease progression, including tobacco use, an unhealthy diet and physical inactivity (which together result in obesity), hypertension, dyslipidaemia and diabetes. Moreover, evidence shows that timely and sustained lifestyle interventions and, when needed, drug treatment will reduce the risk of cardiovascular events, hence reducing premature morbidity, mortality and disability.

Without symptoms, many people are unaware of their risk status. Thus, as with type 2 diabetes, opportunistic screening for individuals at high risk for cardiovascular disease is recommended and a useful means of detecting risk factors, such as raised blood pressure, abnormal blood, lipids and blood glucose.[18] In England a national screening programme was launched in 2009, aimed at people aged between 40 and 74, which offers a free health check to assess cardiovascular disease and diabetes risk, with repeat checks offered every five years (see Table 13.2).

Methods of screening for cardiovascular disease risk

Many guidelines recommend risk assessment for cardiovascular disease for people over 40 years of age, or 10 years earlier for at-risk populations.[20,21] In the past, screening practice focused on protocols for identifying individual risk factors such as elevated blood pressure or cholesterol and defining thresholds for treatment. The development of risk prediction charts, based on combining individual risk factors to estimate total cardiovascular risk, (i.e. the likelihood of a cardiovascular event in the next 5 or 10 years) are a major advance, since they provide a more rational basis for clinical decisions about who should receive treatment, taking account of available resources. There is now a strong body of evidence that this approach can predict an individual's risk of cardiovascular disease with reasonable accuracy across a wide range of countries.[18]

Most risk factor tools are based on a similar set of risk factors and use risk prediction equations derived from epidemiological studies, the most common being the Framingham Heart Study (Table 13.4). The risk charts and tables use different age categories, duration of risk assessment and risk factor profiles. It should be noted that risk scores must be validated within a population and may over-predict in low risk populations and under-predict in high risk populations. More recently, the inclusion of other risk factors, (such as C-reactive protein, fibrinogen, waist-to-hip ratio) to improve accuracy, has been the subject of debate.[18]

Table 13.4 Comparison of cardiovascular disease risk assessment tools

CVD risk tool	Factors	Risk levels
Framingham[21] (risk of a CVD event over 10 years)[18]	Age (20–79 years) Gender Diabetes Smoking Systolic BP TC HDL	Males score: $\geq$12–10% 13–15–20% 16–25% $\geq$17–$\geq$30%
Joint British Societies Guidelines[19] (risk of a CVD event over 10 years)	Age ($<$50, 50–59, $\geq$60 years) Gender Diabetes Smoking Systolic BP TC/HDL ratio	$<$10% – low risk 10–20% – medium risk $>$20% – high risk
NZ risk calculator[20] (5 year risk of a cardiovascular event)	Age (50–65 years) Gender Smoking BP TC/HDL ratio Diabetes	Mild $<$10% Moderate 10–15% High 15–20% Very high – $>$20%
Systematic Coronary Risk Evaluation (SCORE)[22] (10 year risk of a fatal CVD event)	Age (50–65 years) Gender Smoking Systolic BP and either TC or TC/HDL ratio	Threshold for risk of death is 5% or higher
PROCAM[23] (risk of a CVD event over 10 years)	Age (35–65 years) LDL Smoking HDL Systolic BP Family history of premature myocardial infarction Diabetes Triglycerides	Score: 0–20 $<$1% 21–44 $<$10% 45–53 $<$20% 54–61 $<$40%

CVD = cardiovascular disease; TC = total cholesterol; BP = blood pressure; HDL = high density lipoprotein; LDL = low density lipoprotein.

Opportunities for pharmacy screening

The feasibility of screening provision in community pharmacy has been studied in early trials.[24,25] In other cases, pharmacies invited people for lipid screening who were at potential risk, such as those taking antihypertensives, identified from patient medication records.[26] Pharmacists themselves do not necessarily need to undertake the screening, or could also combine it with medication review. In a Canadian study, 30 trained volunteer peer health educators working in community pharmacies assessed 406 older people, of whom 148 (36.5%) had elevated blood pressure, so were referred to the pharmacist and GP for review and follow up.[27] This study and others have demonstrated that pharmacist involvement through review and support positively impacts on adherence to medicines and improved lipid levels.[26]

Research illustrates the feasibility of screening for both cardiovascular disease and diabetes either in community pharmacy or as an outreach service. More importantly there is a valuable opportunity to design pharmacy delivered programmes that combine screening services with health promotion interventions aimed at reducing risk factors in the targeted population. Community pharmacists are being encouraged to provide the national cardiovascular disease screening programme in England, although this service is currently commissioned locally. However, evidence of the clinical and cost-effectiveness as demonstrated through randomised controlled trials is yet to be published.

Evidence for pharmacy screening

Reflecting the evolution of guidelines for cardiovascular disease screening, many early screening trials in community pharmacy focused on individual risk factors such as hypertension[24,26] or dyslipidaemia.[24] Some offered free opportunistic screening to customers visiting the pharmacy, for example, a screening programme for hypertension and stroke in Iowa, USA in 1996. Of the 351 patients screened in this one pharmacy, 216 (62%) were hypertensive, but 103 (29%) had no previous diagnosis.[24] Data from a national survey of Australian pharmacists in 2002 showed much higher numbers of blood pressure tests compared with cholesterol tests (258 282 versus 12 273 tests) over 12 months.

More recently, community pharmacy screening trials have included identifying and referring patients for multiple risk factors, as well as demonstrating efficacy in improving risk factors. For example, a health promotion and screening service for cardiovascular risk factors in nine rural pharmacies in New South Wales, Australia used a risk assessment questionnaire plus measurement of weight, blood pressure, total cholesterol and triglycerides. Over half the 389 people screened had elevated BMI and cholesterol (>5 mmol/L), a fifth had elevated blood pressure (i.e. systolic

≥ 140 mmHg and/or diastolic ≥ 90 mmHg) and participated in less than the recommended level of physical activity. A majority (79%) received lifestyle advice (diet, physical activity, smoking cessation) and over a quarter required GP referral. The programme showed a decrease in mean total cholesterol and mean systolic blood pressure, while a third had increased their physical activity to the recommended level. Overall consumers were very satisfied with the health promotion and screening service offered in community pharmacy.[28]

A trial comparing the effectiveness of screening for cardiovascular disease risk factors involving 888 participants in 26 pharmacies and four non-healthcare settings in Texas found that 81% were referred for follow up for at least one abnormality and of those completing follow up, 16% received one or more new diagnoses and 42% therapy changes. Importantly, pharmacy-based screening achieved higher follow-up rates compared with screening in non-healthcare settings.[16]

Successful pharmacy outreach screening programmes have also been reported. Community pharmacists in Iowa, USA were contracted by two local trade unions to conduct screening for cardiovascular disease risks in their members at the union halls. Pharmacists screened 265 people and calculated 10-year risk for 226 of these. A third had 10–20% risk and 15% had greater than 20% risk with two or more risk factors. This study demonstrated that community pharmacists could identify individuals with intermediate or high 10-year cardiovascular risk and opened up future opportunities for the delivery of pharmacist-led risk management programmes.[29] Another outreach workplace-based programme provided a two-stage screening process for cardiovascular risk factors. Individuals found to be at risk were invited to participate in the Heart Smart programme, which involved a minimum of eight one-to-one education and monitoring sessions with the pharmacist in the first year and six sessions in subsequent years if targets had not been achieved. Of the 96 workers screened, 56 had risk factors for cardiovascular disease and 37 had diabetes. The mean number of visits with the pharmacist was seven, resulting in significant improvements in blood pressure and low density lipoprotein levels.[30]

Cancer

Background

The term cancer represents a group of diseases in which abnormal cells in the body are not destroyed by normal control mechanisms. The result is proliferation and spread of disease. Cancers are defined by the type of cell involved and the place the disease begins. Most cancers, if left untreated, are fatal. However, treatment can either cure a patient or delay death significantly. The success of treatment is related to the type of cancer and its progression. Since treatment is effective in delaying progression of the disease, or eliminating it long term, screening early in the disease process is an important option.

The relative burden of disease, calculated as DALYs, is higher for cancer than for cardiovascular disease in many countries, including the UK and Australia. Prostate is the most common cancer in males and breast in females.[31] Cancer prevalence varies between countries. For example, melanoma prevalence in Australia is particularly high (9.8%) whereas in Canada it is 2.5% and in Japan 0.1%.[31,32] Melanoma incidence has increased more than five-fold in the UK in the past 30 years, particularly in those aged 65 or over. However, breast cancer is in fact the most common form of cancer in the UK, Australia and other developed countries, despite being uncommon in males. Death from cancer, however, is mostly frequently due to lung cancer, with prostate and breast cancers being the second most common. Throughout the world, cancers with the highest five-year survival are testicular (97%), thyroid (93%), melanoma (92%), breast (88%) and prostate (85%).[31]

Although the causes of cancer are many (and yet many other causes are likely still to be identified), by far the major contribution to cancer, measured as attributable risk, is tobacco.[33] Breast cancer risk is increased by breast density and oestradiol,[34] whereas exercise, weight reduction, low fat diet and reduced alcohol intake were associated with a decreased risk of breast cancer. Thus women on hormone replacement therapy and who lead unhealthy lifestyles are likely to be at higher risk. For prostate cancer, risk increases after the age of 50, is higher in some ethnic groups, seems to occur more often in families with an affected member, and may be related to increased red meat consumption. At present there is no association between obesity and lack of exercise and prostate cancer.[32] For cervical cancer, the major risk is human papillomavirus infection (see Chapter 12).[32] Smoking, oral contraceptives over long periods, *Chlamydia* infection and family history also appear to increase risk. For bowel/colon cancer the risks are smoking, high alcohol intake, type 2 diabetes, increased age, family history, eating meat cooked at high temperatures and low intake of fruit and vegetables, as well as low physical activity and obesity.

Methods of screening for cancer

There are four screening programmes currently available. These are for cervical cancer, which uses the Papanicolaou (Pap) test to detect abnormalities in the cervix; breast cancer, which uses mammography; bowel cancer, which uses the faecal occult blood test (FOBT); and prostate cancer, which uses prostate-specific antigen (PSA) levels in the blood. Although screening programmes for the first three cancers are well established and justified, for prostate cancer there is still debate about whether the resources required justify population screening or indeed whether early detection affects mortality.[34,35] Moreover, since not all prostate cancers are aggressive and there is no way of predicting which cancers will remain quiescent, the benefits of early detection and intervention must be weighed against the adverse effects of treatment such as impotence and incontinence.

Availability of screening will depend on resources available. In a review of cost-effectiveness for cancer screening, it was estimated that cost-effectiveness ratios for any current method were between US$10 000 and $25 000 per life-year saved and thus it was considered cost-effective when compared with no screening.[36] Cervical cancer screening costs can be extremely cost-effective for developing countries if the number of screening visits is reduced ($500 per life year saved).

Many countries have issued guidelines for cancer screening programmes that indicate the age groups, recommended tests and their frequency. In the UK, examples of population screening programmes in cancer include the NHS breast screening programme,[37] which targets women aged 50 to 70 for screening every three years and the NHS bowel cancer screening programme,[38] which invites men and women in their 60s to be screened for bowel cancer every two years. Participants are sent an FOBT kit which they complete at home and send to a laboratory. Anyone with a positive result is referred for a colonoscopy and any necessary treatment. Guidelines for cervical screening differ between countries, but in general require that this should be offered to all women initially annually using the regular Pap test, starting about three years after they begin having vaginal intercourse, but no older than 21 and continue at less frequent intervals until about age 70. In general, routine testing for prostate cancer is not advocated at present. Instead, an informed choice programme is in place in the UK, similar to that advocated by the American Cancer Society.[32] Healthcare professionals should discuss the potential benefits and limitations of prostate cancer early detection testing, including offering PSA testing. Only those men who want testing should be tested, but the discussion enables them actively to take part in this decision by learning about prostate cancer and the pros and cons of early detection and treatment.

Opportunities for pharmacy screening

Since the screening programs for cancer are based on population-based screening rather than opportunistic, use of healthcare professionals who have exposure to the general public to increase numbers of those who can be screened is a sensible approach. Community pharmacies are one of the most frequently visited sites where healthcare professionals work, and therefore represent opportunities for screening. It is usual for no costs to be associated with visiting a pharmacy and people often visit when relatively well. It is therefore possible to find and screen people on low incomes who would not visit standard care facilities unless experiencing acute illness.

However, for pharmacists to take on the challenge of community-based screening for cancer, a programme for education and empowerment will be needed. The knowledge base in this area is not a traditional one for pharmacy and a lack of knowledge could be an impediment to involvement.[39] Pharmacists should however, encourage patients and the public to take up screening invitations and be able to explain the benefits of these.

Evidence for pharmacy screening

In a programme in Nebraska, USA, pharmacies enrolled low income patients, who had difficulties in accessing services, in a screening programme for mammography and Pap smears.[40] Patients received a coupon from the pharmacy, which was then delivered to the doctor. Rural pharmacies were much more active and more likely to refer patients even though there was no remuneration involved. In Richmond, Virginia, the breast cancer risk assessment tool, provided by the National Cancer Institute of America, was implemented in six community pharmacies.[41] Pharmacists also provided education and training on breast self examination, clinical examination needs and mammography.

Adherence to guidelines in 140 women increased from 31 to 56%, performance of monthly self examination in high risk women increased from 20 to 60% and the mean number of self examinations increased in 6 months from 2.69 to 4.09%. Thus pharmacist intervention and involvement improved patient-initiated screening.

Other potential areas for pharmacy screening

Screening for mental ill health is an area in which there is great need (see Chapter 11) but one which requires much more evidence. However, sleep disorders have recently been studied[42,43] and a specific pharmacy instrument to screen people at risk of poor sleep health has been developed. Prior to this, screening for poor sleep health was done poorly and of the available instruments, none were valid for the pharmacy setting. Since the Australian study found that 62% of people screened were at risk, the importance of developing this area of screening cannot be underestimated.

Screening for osteoporosis and alcohol overuse are covered in Chapter 11.

Screening within existing conditions and in high risk populations: asthma

Background

Asthma is one of the most common non-communicable diseases in the world and is distinguished by the number of children affected. It has been estimated that 300 million people are affected by the disease.[44] When uncontrolled, it can severely affect a person's life and can be fatal. The current estimate of asthma prevalence varies in different countries. In Australia, 10.2% of the population (adults and children) are affected,[45] while there are an estimated 5.2 million people with asthma in the UK. In the age group of six to seven years, the overall global prevalence is currently 11.5%, ranging from a low of 6.8% in India to 21.7% in Oceania.[46] During the 1980s and 1990s there was a worldwide increase in the prevalence of asthma, which may now have reached a plateau.[47] Whether this rise was due to increased diagnosis or exposure to environmental factors is not clear.

Asthma is an episodic disease, marked by exacerbations and symptom-free periods. It is characterised by episodic shortness of breath, particularly at night, and cough. Factors that may influence the development and expression of asthma include family history, obesity, gender, exposure to allergens, early respiratory infection, tobacco smoke exposure, indoor/outdoor pollution and diet.[4]

Whereas early diagnosis and use of medication can reduce the burden on society, improve quality of life and reduce the risk of dying, the disease cannot be cured. Thus asthma or exacerbations of asthma, can satisfy at least some of the World Health Organization's criteria for screening. There is no preclinical phase that can be recognised by testing and the natural history of the disease is not completely understood.

Although asthma is classified by severity, this may change over time and in response to treatment. It is thus more useful to describe the level of control, which can be described in terms of the need for bronchodilator and the presence of symptoms.[4] In terms of screening, reviewing for these two factors is the most useful method of targeting the burden of disease and need for intervention.

Methods of screening for poor asthma control

Measurement of lung function is recommended as the gold standard since people with asthma often do not perceive their symptoms to be severe. The two lung function measurements currently in use are spirometry and peak expiratory flow measurements. Of these spirometry is the preferred method for diagnosis.[44] Apart from these functional measurements, several instruments can be used to measure asthma control based on patient self report of symptoms. Two commonly used tools are the asthma score[48] and the asthma control questionnaire.[49] A modified version suitable for use by healthcare practitioners has been produced from the Canadian Asthma Consensus conference.[50,51] The level of asthma control should be used to make decisions on need for treatment. This and a similar tool, the Jones morbidity index,[52] have been very useful for screening patients for risk of poorly controlled asthma and have been shown to be sensitive to change after interventions designed to improve control.[53]

Opportunities for pharmacy screening

Pharmacists can easily identify potential patients with asthma whom they care for on a regular basis using patient medication records, to provide a service that screens for poor asthma control. Such an activity is a simple way to get started in a population approach to pharmacy practice.

Evidence for pharmacy screening

Monitoring and screening in community pharmacy has been reviewed previously.[54,55] Spirometry has been used successfully in community pharmacy.[56] Pharmacists given appropriate training can conduct spirometry successfully and screen for poor lung function and lack of optimal disease control.[53] Although they are more likely to refer patients if they have concerns regarding medication and asthma control,[56] they can be trained to take on a more proactive role.[53] It is common for peak expiratory flow measurements to be used as a tool for screening in pharmacy.[54,57–59] This has been shown to be a very useful tool for screening for poor disease management; however, the functional measurements are usually performed by the patient with pharmacists playing a supportive and encouraging role.

Algorithms based on pharmaceutical data have been developed for screening and stratification of asthma patients.[60] This method has the advantage of being able to screen large data sets and has been validated for severity. It does not require input from the pharmacist as such and so could be used in any healthcare setting where the data are available. Questionnaires designed to screen for poor asthma control have also been used in community pharmacy.[52] These instruments can screen for patients at risk in terms of asthma control[53] as well as being sensitive to changes in control following pharmacy interventions.[53,57]

Sale of screening kits from community pharmacies

A number of home testing diagnostic kits are widely available through community pharmacies. There are two types: *test kits* where the patient collects the sample and performs the test or *collection kits* where the sample is collected by the patient and posted to a laboratory. For example, with a cholesterol testing kit clients can measure either total cholesterol only or a full lipid profile including high density lipoprotein cholesterol, low density lipoprotein cholesterol and triglycerides. However, the test results are subject to variability and must also be considered in the context of other risk factors for cardiovascular disease and always discussed with a health professional.

For colon cancer screening, there are currently two different types of FOBT (guaiac and immunochemical) available in the pharmacy. Guaiac tests require patients to alter their diet and medications and require samples from three separate bowel motions. Immunochemical tests are generally more acceptable, as no change to the patient's diet or medication is necessary and samples are only required from two separate bowel motions. Although FOBTs are not the most accurate diagnostic test for bowel cancer, their use is supported by evidence. Currently they are the cheapest and most acceptable method available for population screening.

Although self diagnostic kits are convenient and easy to use, there are strong messages that should be communicated to any purchaser. The test results are subject to the accuracy with which the manufacturer's directions are followed and may therefore be variable. They must never replace a consultation with a healthcare professional. Pharmacists should always serve as a reliable source of information for clients seeking the use of at-home diagnostic test kits. They should assess the client's capacity to perform the test, stress the importance of checking the expiry date, carefully following the manufacturer's directions and ensure that the client understands the proper use of the test.

The future of pharmacy screening

Screening for non-communicable diseases is a public health activity in which pharmacies have a recognised, legitimate and valuable role to play. Proactive involvement in-store or outreach screening programmes linked to follow-up health promotion activities appear to offer the best model for achieving significant impact on population health outcomes. Pharmacists' level of involvement in screening varies widely across countries and settings, with many programmes currently only offered within a research framework. There is undoubtedly significant scope to increase participation in routine pharmacy practice. If pharmacists are to offer these programmes, they must ensure that they meet the requisite professional standards of practice with respect to training, quality assurance of testing equipment and procedures, patient counselling, records, referral and follow up (Box 13.1). Future challenges will focus on further developments in biotechnology and the emergence of new tests for a wide range of conditions. Pharmacy will need to define its role in the implementation of these emerging technologies in screening for undiagnosed disease.

Box 13.1 *International Pharmaceutical Federation professional standards of practice for screening and case detection*[61]

1   Train staff to ensure continuing competency in the use of equipment, standard operating procedures to be followed, risk minimisation, interpretation of results and the limitations of various tests.

2   Institute a quality assurance programme covering equipment and procedures, to ensure the accuracy of results.

3   Retain the results of tests, including full patient details, in an appropriate manner in the pharmacy, complying with all relevant data protection legislation and the profession's code of professional standards in relation to confidentiality.

4   Provide suitable facilities for every aspect of the conduct of the tests, for the segregation, storage and disposal of clinical waste and for dealing with spillage and accidental needle-stick injuries.

5   Ensure that information about the outcome of tests, and appropriate counselling of individuals can be carried out in a location that provides privacy.

6   Work in collaboration with physicians and other professionals providing healthcare to those using the testing services provided in the pharmacy, not least to seek to agree relevant referral criteria.

7   Obtain the informed consent of an individual before carrying out a point of care test which requires the taking of a sample of body fluid and authorisation from individuals, before transmitting the result of a test to any other party, including an individual's physician or other healthcare provider; and in the absence of such authorisation to advise the individual to seek medical advice if the pharmacist considers that to be necessary.

8   Ensure that the professional indemnity insurance held covers all aspects of the provision of the screening and testing service provided.

9   Inform patients with chronic diseases when follow-up tests are required.

References

1. Strong K, Wald N, Miller A *et al.* Group WHOC Current concepts in screening for non-communicable disease: World Health Organization Consultation Group Report on methodology of noncommunicable disease screening. *J Med Screen* 2005; 12(1): 12–19.
2. Braveman PA, Tarim E. *Screening in Primary Health Care: Setting priorities with limited resources.* Geneva: World Health Organization, 1994.
3. Engelau MN, V Herman W. Screening for Type 2 Diabetes. *Diabetes Care* 2000; 23(10): 1563–1580.

4. UK National Screening Committee (homepage). http://www.screening.nhs.uk/about. (accessed 21 October 2009).

5. Australian Institute for Health and Welfare. *Cancer Committees.* Canberra: Australian Institute for Health and Welfare, 2009. http://www.aihw.gov.au/cancer/committees.cfm. (accessed 21 October 2009).

6. International Diabetes Federation. *IDF Diabetes Atlas.* Brussels: IDF, 2009. http://www.eatlas.idf.org/ (accessed 31 July 2009).

7. Engelgau MM, Narayan KM, Herman WH. Screening for type 2 diabetes. *Diabetes Care* 2000; 23(10): 1563–1580.

8. Colagiuri S DD, Girgis S, Colagiuri R. *Evidence Based Guideline for the Case Detection and Diagnosis of Type 2 Diabetes.* Canberra: Diabetes Australia/NHMRC, 2009.

9. Tuomilehto J, Lindstrom J, Eriksson JG *et al.* Prevention of type 2 diabetes mellitus by changes in lifestyle among subjects with impaired glucose tolerance [comment]. *N Engl J Med* 2001; 344: 1343–1350.

10. Diabetes Prevention Reseach Group. Reduction in the incidence of Type 2 diabetes with lifestyle intervention of metformin. *N Engl J Med* 2002; 346: 393–403.

11. American Diabetes Association Screening for diabetes. *Diabetes Care* 2001; 24(Suppl1): 1–9.

12. Krass I, Mitchell B, Clarke P *et al.* Pharmacy diabetes care program: analysis of two screening methods for undiagnosed type 2 diabetes in Australian community pharmacy. *Diabetes Res Clin Pract* 2007; 75(3): 339–347.

13. Berbatis C SB, Mills CR, Bulsara M. *Reference Data Base of Australia's Community Pharmacies: Analysis of national survey.* Perth, WA: Curtin University of Technology, 2003.

14. Simoens S, Foulon E, Dethier M *et al.* Promoting targeted screening for Type 2 diabetes mellitus: the contribution of community pharmacists. *Diabet Med* 2005; 22(6): 812–813.

15. Hersberger KE, Botomino A, Mancini M *et al.* Sequential screening for diabetes–evaluation of a campaign in Swiss community pharmacies. *Pharm World Sci* 2006; 28(3): 171–179.

16. Snella KA, Canales AE, Irons BK *et al.* Pharmacy- and community-based screenings for diabetes and cardiovascular conditions in high-risk individuals. *J Am Pharm Assoc* 2006; 46(3): 370–377.

17. World Health Organization. *Cardiovascular Diseases.* Geneva: WHO, 2009. http://www.who.int/cardiovascular_diseases/en/ (accessed 16 August).

18. World Health Organization. *Prevention of Cardiovascular Disease Guidelines for Assessment and Management of Cardiovascular Risk 2007.* Geneva: WHO, 2007. http://www.who.int/cardiovascular_diseases/guidelines/Full%20text.pdf (accessed 13 August 2009).

19. British Heart Foundation. *Joint British Societies' Guidelines on the Prevention of Cardiovascular Disease in Clinical Practice: Risk assessment.* London: BHF, 2006. http://www.bhf.org.uk/publications/view_publication.aspx?ps=1000349 (accessed 13 August 2009).

20. New Zealand Guidelines Group. *Assessment and Management of Cardiovascular Risk.* Wellington: New Zealand Guidelines Group, 2003. http://www.nzgg.org.nz/guidelines/0035/CVD_Risk_Full.pdf. (accessed 13 August 2009).

21. National Cholesterol Education Program. *ATP III Guidelines At-A-Glance Quick Desk Reference.* Bethesda, MD: US Department of Health and Human services, 2001. http://www.nhlbi.nih.gov/guidelines/cholesterol/atglance.pdf (accessed 13 August, 2009).

22. Conroy RM, Pyorala K, Fitzgerald AP *et al.* Estimation of ten-year risk of fatal cardiovascular disease in Europe: the SCORE project. *Eur Heart J* 2003; 24(11): 987–1003.

23. Assmann G, Cullen P, Schulte H. Simple scoring scheme for calculating the risk of acute coronary events based on the 10-year follow-up of the prospective cardiovascular Munster (PROCAM) study. *Circulation* 2002; 105(3): 310–315.

24. Mangum SA, Kraenow KR, Narducci WA. Identifying at-risk patients through community pharmacy-based hypertension and stroke prevention screening projects. *J Am Pharm Assoc (Wash)* 2003; 43(1): 50–55.

25. McManus RJ, Mant J. Community pharmacies for detection and control of hypertension. *J Hum Hypertens* 2001; 15(8): 509–510.

26. Blenkinsopp A, Anderson C, Armstrong M. Systematic review of the effectiveness of community pharmacy-based interventions to reduce risk behaviours and risk factors for coronary heart disease. *J Public Health Med* 2003; 25(2): 144–153.

27. Jones C, Simpson SH, Mitchell D *et al*. Enhancing hypertension awareness and management in the elderly: lessons learned from the Airdrie Community Hypertension Awareness and Management Program (A-CHAMP). *Can J Cardiol* 2008; 24(7): 561–567.

28. Krass I, Chen TC, Hourihan F. Health promotion and screening for cardiovascular risk factors in NSW: a community pharmacy model. *Aust J Health Prom* 2003; 14(2): 102–108.

29. Liu Y, Mentele LJ, McDonough RP *et al*. Community pharmacist assessment of 10-year risk of coronary heart disease for union workers and their dependents. *J Am Pharm Assoc* 2008; 48(4): 515–517.

30. John EJ, Vavra T, Farris K *et al*. Workplace-based cardiovascular risk management by community pharmacists: impact on blood pressure, lipid levels, and weight. *Pharmacotherapy* 2006; 26(10): 1511–1517.

31. Australian Institute of Health and Welfare. *Cancer in Australia: An overview*. AIHW cat. no. CAN 42 edn. Canberra: AIHW, 2008.

32. American Cancer Society (homepage). Atlanta, GA: ACS. http://www.cancer.org/docroot/home/index.asp (accessed 18 September 2009).

33. National Cancer Institute. *Smoking*. Bethesda, MD: NCI. http://www.cancer.gov/cancertopics/smoking (accessed 18 September 2009).

34. Cummings SR, Tice JA, Bauer S *et al*. Prevention of breast cancer in postmenopausal women: approaches to estimating and reducing risk. *J Natl Cancer Inst* 2009; 101(6): 384–398.

35. Pignone Michael. Weighing the benefits and downsides of prostate-specific antigen screening. *Arch Intern Med* 2009; 169(17): 1554–1556.

36. Pignone M, Saha S, Hoerger T *et al*. Cost-effectiveness analyses of colorectal cancer screening: a systematic review for the US Preventive Services Task Force. *Ann Intern Med* 2002; 137(2): 96–104.

37. UK National Screeening Committee. *NHS Breast Screening Programme*. London: UK National Screeening Committee, 2009. http://www.screening.nhs.uk/breastcancer-england (accessed 21 October, 2009).

38. UK National Screeening Committee. *NHS Bowel Cancer Screening Programmes*. London: UK National Screeening Committee, 2009. http://www.screening.nhs.uk/bowelcancer-england (accessed 21 October 2009).

39. Odedina FT, Warrick C, Vilme H *et al*. Pharmacists as health educators and risk communicators in the early detection of prostate cancer. *Res Soc Admin Pharm* 2008; 4(1): 59–66.

40. McGuire TR, Leypoldt M, Narducci WA *et al*. Accessing rural populations: role of the community pharmacist in a breast and cervical cancer screening programme. *J Eval Clin Pract* 2007; 13(1): 146–149.

41. Giles JT, Kennedy DT, Dunn EC *et al*. Results of a community pharmacy-based breast cancer risk-assessment and education program. *Pharmacotherapy* 2001; 21(2): 243–253.

42. Hersberger KE, Renggli VP, Nirkko AC *et al*. Screening for sleep disorders in community pharmacies: evaluation of a campaign in Switzerland. *J Clin Pharm Ther* 2006; 31(1): 35–41.

43. Tran A, Fuller J, Wong K *et al*. The development of a sleep disorder screening program in Australian community pharmacies. *Pharm World Sci* 2009; 31(4): 473–480.

44. Global Initiative for Asthma. *Global Strategy for Asthma Management and Prevention* (updated 2008). GINA, 2006. http://www.ginasthma.org/ (accessed 18 September 2009).

45. Australian Institute of Health and Welfare. *Asthma in Australia*. Canberra: AIHW, 2008.

46. Lai CKW, Beasley R, Crane J *et al*. Global variation in the prevalence and severity of asthma symptoms: Phase Three of the International Study of Asthma and Allergies in Childhood (ISAAC). *Thorax* 2009; 64(6): 476–483.

47. Asher MI, Montefort S, Björkstén B *et al*. Worldwide time trends in the prevalence of symptoms of asthma, allergic rhinoconjunctivitis, and eczema in childhood: ISAAC Phases One and Three repeat multicountry cross-sectional surveys. *Lancet* 2006; 368(9537): 733–743.

48. Anon. *Asthma Score*. https://www.asthmascore.com.au/ (accessed 18 September 2009).

49. Juniper EF, Buist AS, Cox FM *et al*. Validation of a standardized version of the asthma Quality of Life Questionnaire. *Chest* 1999; 115: 1265–1270.

50. Ernst P, Fitzgerald JM, Spier S. Canadian Asthma Consensus Conference: summary of recommendations. *Can Respir J* 1996; 3(2): 89–101.

51. National Asthma Council Australia. *Asthma Management Handbook*. Melbourne, Vic.: NACA, 2006: http://www.nationalasthma.org.au/cms/index.php.

52. Nishiyama T, Chrystyn H. The Jones Morbidity Index as an aid for community pharmacists to identify poor asthma control during the dispensing process. *Int J Pharm Pract* 2003; 11: 41–46.

53. Armour C, Bosnic-Anticevich S, Brillant M *et al*. Pharmacy Asthma Care Program (PACP) improves outcomes for patients in the community. *Thorax* 2007; 62(6): 496–592.

54. Armour CL, Smith L, Krass I. Community pharmacy, disease state management, and adherence to medication: a review. *Dis Manage Health Outcomes* 2008; 16(4): 245–254.

55. Armour C, Saini B, Bosnic-Anticevich S *et al*. Roles of pharmacists in asthma monitoring: monitoring asthma. In: Gibson P, ed. *Lung Biology in Health and Disease*. Boca Raton, FL: Taylor & Francis, 2005: 465–502.

56. Simpson M, Burton D, Burton M *et al*. Impact of spirometry on pharmacists' decision to refer. *Aust Pharm* 2005; 24(12): 964–968.

57. Saini B, Krass I, Armour C. Development, implementation, and evaluation of a community pharmacy-based asthma care model. *Ann Pharmacother* 2004; 38(11): 1954–1960.

58. Bheekie A, Syce J, Weinberg E. An assessment of asthmatic patients at far Western Cape community pharmacies. *S Afr Med J* 1998; 88: 1998; 262–266.

59. Bheekie A, Syce JA, Weinberg EG. Peak expiratory flow rate and symptom self-monitoring of asthma initiated from community pharmacies. *J Clin Pharm Ther* 2001; 26(4): 287–296.

60. Leone FT, Grana JR, McDermott P *et al*. Pharmaceutically-based severity stratification of an asthmatic population. *Respir Med* 1999; 93(11): 788–793.

61. International Pharmaceutical Federation. *FIP Statement of Policy Point of Care Testing in Pharmacies*. The Hague: IPF, 2004. http://www.fip.org/statements (accessed 21st September 2009).

14

Medicines management

Janet Krska and Brian Godman

There is no widely accepted definition of medicines management, although the term is widely used. The National Prescribing Centre in England defines it as: 'a system of processes and behaviours that determines how medicines are used by patients and by the NHS.'[1] When first described in 2002, medicines management encompassed clinical assessment, monitoring and review in individual patients, medicines delivery services, review of repeat prescribing systems, clinical audit, health education, risk management, disease prevention and formularies and guidelines. Some of these topics are covered elsewhere in this book. Recent developments in the UK have resulted in considerable changes in the ways medicines are used, hence medicines management has also changed. These important developments include non-medical prescribing, increasing clinical roles of community pharmacists, changes in the way that GPs and pharmacists are remunerated for their NHS work, electronic prescribing, early discharge from hospital, hospital at home services, minor ailments services, pharmacy public health services and more standards for care quality. Similar changes are going on in many countries.

Many medicines management activities as listed above are aimed at individuals. However, many are also targeted at populations and are designed to improve the overall health of a population, hence form part of public health. This chapter focuses on these activities, in particular, tools for managing, monitoring and improving the use of medicines in populations, such as formularies, guidelines and prescribing indicators, which are similar in many countries. These topics consider the cost-effective use of medicines, which form part of public health activities related to health and social care (clinical effectiveness) (see Box 1.1) Safety of medicines in use is just as important and forms part of health protection (Box 1.1). Key public health activities here are policies on safe handling of medicines, pharmacovigilance and risk management.

Ensuring cost-effective use of medicines within populations

Everywhere in the world, purchasing and supplying medicines (often regarded as pharmacists' core function) constitutes a major component of health costs. In the UK, as in many European countries, pharmaceutical expenditure is already or is approaching the largest cost component of healthcare. Pharmaceutical expenditure is set to rise more rapidly than other components unless addressed.[2] The reasons for this are well known and include demographic changes leading to greater prevalence of chronic diseases, rising patient expectations, stricter clinical targets and the continued launch of new premium priced products. Resources are however, finite and there is a need to maximise the efficiency with which medicines are utilised as a resource. The World Health Organization emphasises the need for rational prescribing, which is based on efficacy, safety, patient acceptability and cost.[3] To ensure rational prescribing, both prescribers and patients need to be aware of why this is beneficial. However, in practice, medicines are frequently not prescribed appropriately or used appropriately by patients. Many reports from various sources have stated that that improvements in prescribing are possible, which could improve cost-effectiveness without compromising efficacy.[3,4] Improving the use of medicines in individuals also has the potential to improve cost-effectiveness, by reducing waste and improving health outcomes, including minimising adverse drug reactions and drug–drug interactions. All require interventions designed to influence behaviour, in both health professionals and patients. The main strategies currently used to achieve this can be described as the 'four Es': education, engineering, economics and enforcement.[5] Examples of these are given in Table 14.1.

Although all have strengths and may help to rationalise prescribing, they often have weaknesses too. For example, the extent to which clinical guidance is followed may be variable and the pharmaceutical industry will seek alternative ways to influence prescribers, since this is necessary for industry to achieve increased sales, just as clinicians will seek ways to get around restrictions on prescribing. Initiatives designed to improve patients' use of medicines are usually targeted at individuals, although the strategic provision of such services forms part of the overall medicines management approach to rationalising medicines use.

Tools for influencing prescribing

Pharmacists have, for many years, been instrumental in developing tools for reducing the range of drugs prescribed and assisting in implementing these in practice.[6] A variety of tools, policies and incentives are used in many countries

Table 14.1 Examples of the 'four E' approach to influencing prescribing

Measure	Methods	Examples
Education	Distribute guidelines	NICE clinical guidelines
	Educational outreach visits	Practice-based pharmacist activities
	Public campaigns	Campaign on antibiotics for viral infections
Engineering	Setting prescribing targets	Prescribing quality indicators
	Formulary management systems	Limiting pharmaceutical company representative activities
Economics	Incentive schemes	Payments for non-dispensing
	Payment methods	Quality and outcomes framework (QOF)
Enforcement	Generic substitution	Contract purchasing in secondary care
	Restrictions on prescribing	Authorisation to prescribe non-formulary medicines

Adapted from reference 5.

to try to influence prescribing. The three main tools which pharmacists routinely use for improving prescribing are:

- formularies, which recommend specific drugs and exclude others
- clinical guidelines, which help to ensure that treatment of patients is based on evidence of best practice
- prescribing policies/treatment protocols, which assist prescribers in using the drugs in a formulary or implementing clinical guidelines.

Used together, formularies, clinical guidelines and treatment policies/protocols can ensure that standards of prescribing are uniform, high quality and cost-effective and there are many of these tools available. Internationally, many countries have, often with the technical advice of the World Health Organization, produced essential medicines lists and national treatment guidelines. These frequently include information about how to use medicines and are particularly important in developing countries, since this provides information for local health workers, who may not always be highly qualified and procurement of medicines can focus around the essential medicines lists.[7]

At a national level within the UK, NICE, Scottish Intercollegiate Guidelines Network (SIGN), the All Wales Medicines Strategy Group and the Scottish Medicines Consortium (SMC) provide advice, guidelines and directions. In addition, various groups such as Royal Colleges produce guidelines for national use. Individual medicines are approved for NHS use in

Scotland by the SMC, so prescribing of those not approved is regularly questioned. To achieve this, SMC reviews all new products shortly after marketing. There is currently no similar process in England, however, NICE issues single or multiple technology appraisals. These cover medicines, as well as other technologies, usually involving novel products for conditions with a high disease burden or high cost or policy implications or when there is evidence of variation in availability or use of the medicines across the country. If medicines are recommended by a NICE technology appraisal, the NHS is then legally obliged to fund them.

Many other regional or local health organisations are also involved in providing guidance. For example, in the UK, regional health organisations may have priority setting committees, PCTs may have area prescribing committees (APCs), hospitals have drug and therapeutics committees (DTCs), all of which provide more local formularies and guidance. Even more specific formularies and policies may be produced by individual departments/wards and general practices.

Other European countries have adopted similar approaches. In Austria, a 'medicines and reasons' initiative was introduced in 1999 to enhance rational prescribing, through the production and dissemination of one guideline per year, which are well accepted and have impacted positively on prescribing.[8] Pharmacists are involved in the production of these and patient versions are available in community pharmacies. Pharmacist involvement in Swedish formularies and guidance extends to monitoring drug utilisation and providing educational input.[9] In France, 243 guidelines were introduced between 1994 and 1999 which included penalties for non-compliance. However, the large number produced resulted in limited awareness among physicians, who were reluctant to implement these guidelines.[10] Subsequently, specific campaigns using guidelines targeted towards improving prescribing for selected groups of drugs have begun to influence prescribing.

Much effort goes into the development, production and distribution of these tools, which aim to achieve standardisation in healthcare provision. In general most are based on evidence (see Chapter 7) and some have considerable ownership among the stakeholders expected to use them, which is an essential component of effective guidance. Their effectiveness in influencing prescribing is however, variable. There is little robust evidence of the benefits of formularies in the form of randomised controlled trials.[11] However, controlled studies have shown that active promotion of a formulary can both change prescribing behaviour and prevent rising drug expenditure.[6,8,11] In addition, a recent ecological study conducted in Sweden studied the association between surrogate markers for hypertension, diabetes and hypercholesterolaemia and adherence to formulary drugs.[12] This study found that although there were no significant associations between adherence and outcomes, following guidelines did results in significant cost savings.

Formularies

A formulary is a list of drugs/medicinal products recommended for use and available for use in a given population.[13] It needs to be owned by those required to prescribe from it, hence representatives of all prescribers need to have input into its development and it must be regularly revised to keep it up to date. Increasingly local formularies are developed for joint use between primary and secondary care, since these facilitate better continuity of care. A formulary management system is usually needed to initiate, develop, monitor, manage and review a local formulary and any prescribing policies contained within it. Key factors in this system are the mechanisms for including new products and deleting products, changes in indication, processes for prescribing of non-formulary medicines and monitoring of adherence to the formulary.

Use of a restricted medicines list is influenced by the number of medicines it contains. To ensure adherence, regular reminders of the restricted range of medicines selected are important, as is feedback on their use. Feedback on adherence should provide information about the cost implications of non-adherence, plus percentage of non-formulary medicines prescribed. As with other prescribing information, such feedback is particularly useful when comparisons with peer groups are included. It is facilitated by computerised prescribing data and likely to be enhanced by educational, face-to-face delivery.[5,6,13] Health organisations may also provide financial incentives to encourage prescribing of approved products.[5,10,14]

Guidelines

A clinical guideline is 'a series of systematically developed statements to assist practitioner and patient decisions about appropriate healthcare for specific clinical circumstances'.[15] Guidelines may not indicate which specific drug or product to use in any given circumstance, often recommending a therapeutic class. Smaller local groups such as DTCs may develop their own guidelines or adapt national guidelines for local use. In developing guidelines, the strength of the evidence, derived from critical appraisal of the design and quality of the studies, influences the grade of the recommendations made. This therefore differentiates those based on strong evidence from those based on weaker evidence, providing an indication of the likelihood that the predicted outcome will be achieved if a recommendation is implemented. Guideline users must be able to form an opinion about how the guideline was developed, and international consensus is available on best practice in guideline development (Box 14.1).[16]

Prescribing policies

Prescribing policies are more detailed than a formulary, giving details of medicines which should be selected for use in specific medical conditions, but are not as wide ranging in scope as clinical guidelines. Important prescribing policies designed to protect health include antibiotic policies, head lice

Box 14.1 *AGREE II (Appraisal of Guidelines for Research and Evaluation) criteria for appraising clinical guideline*[16]*

Scope and purpose

1   The overall objective(s) of the guideline should be specifically described.
2   The clinical question(s) covered by the guideline should be specifically described.
3   The patients to whom the guideline is meant to apply should be specifically described.

Stakeholder involvement

4   The guideline development group should include individuals from all the relevant professional groups.
5   The patients' views and preferences should be sought.
6   The target users of the guideline are clearly defined.
7   The guideline has been piloted among target users.

Rigour of development

8   Systematic methods should be used to search for evidence.
9   The criteria for selecting the evidence should be clearly described.
10   The methods used for formulating the recommendations should be clearly described.
11   The health benefits, side effects and risks should be considered in formulating the recommendations.
12   There should be an explicit link between the recommendations and the supporting evidence.
13   The guideline should be externally reviewed by experts prior to publication.
14   A procedure for updating the guideline should be provided.

Clarity and presentation

15   The recommendations should be specific and unambiguous.
16   The different options for management of the condition should be clearly presented.
17   Key recommendations should be easily identifiable.
18   The guideline should be supported with tools for application.

Applicability

19   The potential organizational barriers in applying the recommendations should be discussed.

20 The potential cost implications of applying the recommendations should be considered.

21 The guideline should present key review criteria for monitoring and audit purposes.

Editorial independence

22 The guideline should be editorially independent from the funding body.

23 Conflicts of interest of guideline development members should be recorded.

*Items from the AGREE Instrument are kindly reproduced with permission from the AGREE Research Trust (www.agreetrust.org).

eradication policies and malarial prophylaxis policies. Treatment protocols go even further in that they specify exactly what should happen to patients throughout their journey of care. This can involve information about diagnosis, processes for recall and review, investigations, detailed instructions about prescribing, non-drug treatments, monitoring, recording and information requirements.

Tools for monitoring prescribing

Methods of assessing how medicines are used are numerous, but those most commonly used include analysis of prescribing data, drug utilisation reviews, prescribing indicators and clinical audit. These require differing levels of effort and the value of the data they provide may reflect that effort. One may lead to another, for example, analysis of prescribing data or a prescribing indicator may provide a prompt to investigate a particular area further using clinical audit.

Studying patterns of medicines use requires data acquired from measures of drug purchase, drug distribution or prescriptions. Evaluating medicines use, also known as drug use evaluation, involves assessing the appropriateness of prescribing and the outcomes achieved, so requires more detailed data which can be derived from medical records or patients. Either can be carried out in specific contexts, such as in a single general practice or a hospital ward, a clinical condition or a particular group of patients.

Monitoring activities often assume some form of standards, against which practice is evaluated, such as a formulary, guidelines or prescribing indicator. As with formularies, increasingly monitoring of indicators is linked to financial incentives and payment. For example, in the UK, GPs income for providing NHS services is in part calculated using a quality and outcomes framework (QOF).[17] This identifies standards of good clinical practice, covering important diseases, but also good management practice, including how medicines are prescribed. Some examples of QOF indicators are given in Table 14.2. Another example is found in Sweden where two indicators are used. These are the number of different drugs prescribed by an individual GP and the overall adherence to the recommended prescribing guidance measured as the proportion of recommend drugs among those drugs accounting for 90% of prescribed volumes in defined daily doses (DDDs – see page 253).[9,14]

Table 14.2 Examples of indicators taken from various sources

Indicator	Unit	Source
Generic prescribing for drug items (i.e. BNF Chapters 1–15)	Percentage	Audit commission
Benzodiazepines	ADQs per STAR-PU	Audit commission
Ulcer healing drugs	ADQs per STAR-PU	Prescribing indicator group
Prescribing rates of antibacterial drugs	Items per STAR-PU	Healthcare commission
Prescribing of low cost statins	Percentage of items of low cost statins (simvastatin and pravastatin) compared with all items for statins, excluding combinations with ezetimibe	Better care, better value indicators
Patients with non-haemorrhagic stroke or TIA taking aspirin, other antiplatelet drug or anticoagulant (unless contraindication recorded)	Percentage of total registered patients with condition	QOF
Patients with diabetes immunised against influenza in preceding winter	Percentage of total registered patients with condition	QOF

TIA = transient ischaemic attack; ADQ = average daily quantity; QOF = quality and outcomes framework.

Monitoring prescribing is not simply an end in itself, but a means of identifying actions to improve prescribing. A wide variety of information sources are used in monitoring medicines use. These include medicines distribution data, prescribing data, patient medication records within community pharmacies and medical records. Analysing prescribing data can show trends over time, illustrate the impact of changes in availability or highlight unexplained variation between groups of prescribers or between populations. The subsequent activities undertaken to address these issues may include clinical medication review, a lower level of review such as medicine use review or prescription review, therapeutic switching programmes, clinical audit, drug utilisation reviews and drug use evaluation.

A variety of numerators and denominators have been developed to enable comparisons in prescribing patterns to be made over time and between populations. International systems for classifying drugs (the anatomical therapeutic chemical system (ATC)), and for quantifying drug use (the defined daily dose (DDD)) have facilitated such comparisons. A DDD is available for every drug on the market, based on the average recommended daily maintenance dose for the drug when used for its most common indication in adults. DDDs are often used as a numerator in prescribing analysis. More sophisticated methods of quantifying prescribing data are also used in the UK primary care setting. The 'average daily quantity' has been developed for a number of drugs to reflect typical prescribing in England. Data can also be expressed in terms of cost, rather than quantity.

The most commonly used denominator is 1000 patients. For example, the DDD of diazepam is 10 mg. If used with a DDD of 2000/1000/year, this means that for every 1000 people, 2000 doses of diazepam were prescribed in a year, equivalent to two doses per person per year. Often DDDs per thousand inhabitants per day is used as a standard quantity: DDD/TID. The use of DDDs enables account to be taken of quantities prescribed and frequency of administration. Using a denominator that takes account of the differing needs of populations enhances this further. Examples of this are the ASTRO-PU (which accounts for the age, sex and temporary residential status of a population) and the STAR-PU which also accounts for variability within therapeutic groups.

Data are used to enable identification of prescribing that is higher or lower than the 'norm' for the actual population served, either in terms of quantity and cost. It is important to use other data to support analysis of prescribing data, to ensure that possible reasons for deviation from 'norms' are considered. For example, in an area with higher than usual prevalence of cardiovascular disease, higher than average levels of prescribing of relevant medicines would be expected, indeed encouraged. It is also important to recognise that average prescribing can still be below or above the 'norm' if disease prevalence deviates substantially from average.

Prescribing indicators

Prescribing indicators are quantitative measures of prescribing that can be used to estimate the quality of prescribing and again enable comparisons to be made between prescribers, regions and countries. One of the main ways in which prescribing indictors are used is to enable peer pressure to influence prescribers' behaviour, such that they are encouraged to work towards the average or norm of prescribing. The applicability of indicators must be reviewed regularly, as new medicines become available and opinions about what constitutes 'high quality prescribing' change with emerging evidence. Other factors that may influence the applicability of an indicator are improvements in performance over time (for example, in the proportion of patients prescribed aspirin for secondary prevention of cardiovascular events), new drugs that may supersede older ones and changes in morbidity within the population. A variety of indicators have been developed which are used nationally in England to assess the quality of prescribing. Some examples of these are given in Table 14.2. Similar indicators, especially those that focus on the prescribing of low cost alternatives versus premium priced, single sourced products in a class or related classes, are also used in other European countries.[9,10]

Using the basic variables outlined above, simple indicators such as the number of prescriptions for isosorbide mononitrate modified release per 1000 adjusted population can illustrate the extent to which these premium priced products are being used. Minimising the prescribing of such products and replacing them with generically prescribed standard release products enables therapeutic goals to be achieved while reducing costs. Having identified an issue such as this, pharmacists may develop a programme to switch patients on to the cheaper alternative and subsequently to monitor any change achieved using the same indicators. Indicators can also be used to identify areas where education or policy development may be needed, such as those relating to antibiotics. However, evaluating the effect of such programmes or developments requires intensive effort to collect data from the records of patients actually prescribed these drugs. Prescribing indicators can provide some data about whether prescribing practices have changed, but they are simply derived from information about what has been prescribed, not why. In other words prescribing indicators lack any association with clinical data, such as diagnosis, co-morbidity and response to the medicine prescribed. Therefore, although they may have been agreed by 'experts' as indicators of prescribing quality, their use does have limitations. As computerisation of medical records increases, the ease with which clinical data can be captured routinely increases. This enables more realistic indicators of quality prescribing to be developed and tested, which incorporate diagnosis and monitoring (see Table 14.2). Indeed the QOF has also resulted in a substantial increase in routine recording of indicators of quality medical practice, many of which include prescribing.

Ensuring high quality prescribing

One of the main ways of improving the quality of prescribing is to ensure that all the formularies, guidance and policies, developed with so much effort, are followed. NICE provides a range of tools to help with implementing its guidance.[18,19] Interventions which are mostly effective include reminders, education outreach (also known as academic detailing) and interactive educational workshops.[6] Simple audit and feedback, use of opinion leaders, local consensus conferences and patient-mediated interventions are less effective.[15] However, multiple or multi-faceted interventions are probably most effective.[6,9,15]

Review of repeat prescribing

In the UK, a system has developed in medical practices to enable patients requiring regular medicines to obtain a prescription without the need to see a doctor, the repeat prescribing system. This is so extensive that around 75% of all prescriptions written are repeats, which are generated by staff using computer systems. The repeat prescribing system is made up of three components: production, management control and clinical control.[20] There is though evidence that repeat prescribing systems are not effectively controlled, resulting in patients requesting items unnecessarily and inappropriately. Consequently, systems should be regularly assessed to ensure that effective controls are in place to minimise the risk of this occurring.[21]

Further developments in primary care within the UK and elsewhere include electronic transfer of prescriptions between medical practices and community pharmacies and repeat dispensing systems. In the latter system, the repeat prescription is valid for several months and the pharmacist is responsible for ensuring continued need, efficacy and safety of each drug at every dispensing. This provides pharmacists with an opportunity to exercise some clinical control over repeat prescribing since they should be seeing patients regularly. It may be appropriate for a pharmacist to undertake a more substantial review of an individual patient's medicines periodically and a nationally agreed service is now increasingly provided by community pharmacists, the medicine use review service.

At an individual level, repeat dispensing and medicine use reviews can help to minimise inappropriate medicines use and reduce waste. Clinical medication reviews, using medical records, and clinical audit activities can help to implement evidence-based formularies and guidelines. Pharmacists frequently provide these services, but GPs and nurses also review patients' medicines, and increasingly so since the introduction of medication review standards in the QOF in the UK. QOF standards relate to specific conditions, but also to patients taking repeat medicines, hence could include medicine use review and holistic clinical reviews. Pharmacists could be involved in developing templates for GPs and nurses to use and in training them in review techniques to improve the quality of reviews in the overall population.[22,23]

Therapeutic switching programmes

As highlighted above, ensuring cost-effective and evidence-based prescribing may involve changing patients from one medicine to another. When carried out for a population, this has become known as a switch. Switches may be of varying types, including:

- changes to generic medicine
- changes to a different drug within the therapeutic group, e.g. proton pump inhibitors or statins, to reduce costs

- changes to the dose, e.g. from a treatment dose of proton pump inhibitors to a maintenance dose
- changes to the formulation, e.g. from dry powder inhaler to a metered dose inhaler
- changes to the formulation and dose, e.g. from modified release to standard diclofenac
- changes to the product because of lack of efficacy, e.g. from a topical non-steroidal anti-inflammatory drug to a rubifacient.

Usually such switches are done using medical records but without seeing the patient. A systematic method of carrying out this activity is required. An example is shown in Box 14.2.

In hospitals, generic prescribing is encouraged, but regardless of whether brand or generic names are used, only one brand of a particular medicine is usually stocked. Switching to generic prescribing in primary care, however, has resulted in large cost savings and the proportion of generic prescribing is in fact a prescribing indicator (see Table 14.2). There is currently the possibility of generic substitution being permitted in primary care in England, which may

---

Box 14.2 *Example of processes required for a therapeutic switching programme*

- Decide on criteria for including patients in the switch and exclusions.
- Ensure community pharmacists are aware of plans to ensure adequate stocks and minimise waste.
- Identify all patients prescribed relevant product.
- Identify who initiated product.
- Review medical records to determine suitability for switching products.
- Confirm with community pharmacist product being dispensed.
- Confirm that appropriate monitoring is being carried out.
- Draft letter to be sent to patients and either attach to next prescription or send by post.
- Contact patients by telephone to confirm their use of the product and receipt of letter.
- Document the switch in records.
- Make changes to repeat prescriptions.
- Record any responses from patients and reasons for reverting back to original product.
- Assess effectiveness of switching protocol by measuring proportion of successful switches.

have the potential for further savings although, of course, for some medicines there is a need for brand retention in individual patients, and the risk of differing adverse reaction profiles caused by varying excipients must not be forgotten.

Managing high cost medicines

Increasingly new medicines are often expensive and well publicised to the public, particularly if they involve major therapeutic advances. Often they require specialist medical knowledge to use effectively and as such may be initiated in secondary care. The introduction of a novel, expensive product can easily put pressure on a restricted prescribing budget, therefore managing this becomes an imperative. Indeed, the continued introduction of new, premium priced drugs is seen as the biggest threat to continued and comprehensive healthcare in Europe.[2] Systems need to be in place to ensure that prescribing of high cost products is controlled and budgeted for, but such systems must also ensure equity of access for patients.[2] This is already happening in the UK and other European countries. Although often initiated in hospitals, where long term use is required, ultimately these products will be prescribed in primary care settings. If not managed properly, with clear financial accountability agreed, tensions can arise between the acute and primary care providers especially following budget devolution. For some products, guidance is available from NICE on when they should be used. For all such technology appraisals, NICE also produces costing tools to enable the calculation of the likely financial impact of the product's introduction.[24] This information can be used to estimate costs locally, based on data derived from the local population. The National Prescribing Centre also produces information on the likely budget impact of new products in primary care. Other national organisations produce information for use in the other home countries.

One consequence of the escalating cost of medicines and the need to restrict availability of high cost products is frequently highlighted by the media, as 'postcode prescribing'. This is the apparent inequitable access to medicines arising when one locality or hospital approves a product for use which a neighbouring locality or hospital does not. It is essential that robust, processes are in place so that any decisions about whether or not to fund individual high cost products are consistent, rational and defensible. The DoH has produced guidance on the processes which should be in place to support decision making about medicines availability.[25,26]

Area prescribing committees

It is clear from the above that patients may obtain different medicines from various sources at different times; some may be supplied by community pharmacists, others by secondary care. Furthermore they may require support with medicines taking from a wider range of services, including social care. It is therefore essential that medicines provision and support are coordinated. Area prescribing committees bring together representatives from all local organisations which have a role in managing medicines. Their role as described by the National Prescribing Centre[27] includes 'coordinating the safe and cost-effective use of medicines across a health community to improve outcomes for patients'. It is often the committee that makes decisions about which medicines to fund locally. Other functions that may be carried out by the committee with the potential to affect the quality of prescribing are: identifying the need for and/or developing shared care protocols and treatment guidelines, contributing to 'traffic light' systems for shared care (see page 259), developing formularies and local guidance, developing incentive schemes, providing guidance on working with the pharmaceutical industry and facilitating public campaigns.

Ensuring safe use of medicines within populations

Role of the National Patient Safety Agency

As described in Chapter 10, the NPSA, a special health authority of the NHS, created in 2001, plays a very important role in minimising the risks associated with medicines supply and administration. As well as coordinating learning from errors, the NPSA issues alerts that are designed to ensure that appropriate action is taken when safety issues with medicines become apparent through this system. An example is *Safer Lithium Therapy*, which was issued in December 2009,[28] requesting healthcare organisations to ensure that patients are monitored in accordance with NICE guidance, results of monitoring are shared appropriately, patients receive all relevant information, and systems are in place to identify and address use of interacting medicines. Alerts such as this also carry a date by which time organisations are expected to have implemented the guidance, in this case, 31 December 2010. To support this, the NPSA produce information leaflets and booklets for patients to record their serum lithium levels.

Medicines safety across the interface

When patients move from one healthcare setting to another, or between healthcare and other settings, information about their medicines needs to move with them. There are many situations when this does not occur and a proportion of these can result in harm. An example of this is the failure to reconcile medicines prescribed on hospital admission with those being taken prior to the admission. The NPSA and NICE issued a joint alert in December 2007, requiring pharmacists to be involved in medicines reconciliation as soon as possible after admission, with all staff having clear responsibilities about obtaining information to facilitate this.[29] Hence policies and procedures must be developed to ensure that these requirements are achieved. This may be undertaken by multi-disciplinary staff working together in the individual hospital. However, in general, it is an APC or DTC which has responsibility for ensuring that NPSA alerts are implemented locally.

Clearly discharge from hospital is another situation where errors can occur with medicines. Indeed, a recent report by the Care Quality Commission indicated that 81% of GP practices surveyed reported that details of medicines prescribed by hospitals were incomplete or inaccurate all or most of the time.[30] From April 2010, all NHS trusts in England are required by law to register with the Commission and must meet standards, including effective medicines management, as a requirement of registration. Electronic discharge summaries, populated with patient and medication information from electronic prescribing systems, have the potential to reduce errors occurring through transcription or illegibility.[31] These can be transmitted electronically to GPs, reducing delays, but obviously a clinical check will still be required to ensure that all medicines are in fact required after discharge. Another initiative with the potential to reduce problems is the Summary Care Record, which has been piloted in several areas of England. This is an electronic record which is web-based, but very securely protected and can thus be accessed by any health professional providing care to an individual patient, with the patient's permission.[32]

For some medicines, safety concerns arise because of their inherent toxicity or the need for invasive monitoring, resulting in the need for continued secondary care involvement in prescribing. Sometimes prescribing may also be restricted to initiating and continuing supply by hospital clinicians only for other reasons. Such medicines often require a shared care approach to prescribing, since patients will almost inevitably be resident in the community most of the time and may be highly inconvenienced by the need for frequent hospital visits to obtain medicines supplies. Shared care protocols are routinely developed for medicines such as these and others, usually by an APC. Many areas use a 'traffic light system' to classify medicines which are used entirely by secondary care specialists (red), those which require shared care and may need a specific protocol (amber) and those which are prescribed freely (green). They may also highlight medicines which are not recommended at all, because of lack of evidence of efficacy, or no benefits over other therapies. Hence the system also supports the local formulary. Several examples are available via the internet.

Medicines safety in non-healthcare settings.

Wherever people live or spend time, they may use medicines, for example, in care homes, prisons, respite care or schools. In these situations, staff are not trained health professionals but may be involved in administering or advising people about how to use their medicines. Therefore safety can only be assured by having policies and procedures in place to manage medicines properly. Safe and secure handling policies are frequently developed by pharmacists or by the local APC/DTC for use in these settings. Care homes are regularly inspected by the Care Quality Commission and medicines policies and practices are an important aspect of this inspection. The RPSGB has produced guidance for the safe handling of medicines in care settings.[33]

Controlled drugs

The Care Quality Commission is also responsible for assessing and overseeing how health and social care providers manage controlled drugs.[34] The Commission, together with a wide range of organisations, are involved in managing controlled drugs to ensure their safety in use (Figure 14.1).

The Commission maintains a register of accountable officers, who are employees of NHS organisations or private hospitals, with designated responsibility for ensuring that safe systems are in place for managing and using controlled drugs. These officers are often pharmacists. Another of their responsibilities is to establish local intelligence networks involving all the key local organisations with involvement in controlled drug use to enable information to be shared. This facilitates appropriate action in the event of incidents involving these drugs.

Pharmacovigilance

Pharmacovigilance is defined by the World Health Organization as the 'science and activities relating to the detection, assessment, understanding and prevention of adverse effects or any other possible drug-related problems'. The need for continuous pharmacovigilance arises because of the nature of pre-marketing requirements for medicines, which frequently involve short term studies, in relatively small number of patients who may be highly selected. Indeed clinical trials are capable of identifying only type A adverse drug reactions (ADRs) (predictable by the pharmacological action of the drug) that affect 1 in 250 or more patients studied. After marketing, medicines will subsequently be used in much larger populations, with characteristics often unlike those included in pre-marketing studies such as greater co-morbidity, and for longer periods of time. Hence the opportunity for ADRs to develop is increased, particularly those that have a long latency, are rare or involve interaction with other medicines or conditions.

ADRs are a major public health problem, estimated to be between the fourth and sixth leading cause of death in the USA and a source of cost to healthcare providers. A large UK cross-sectional study estimated that ADRs

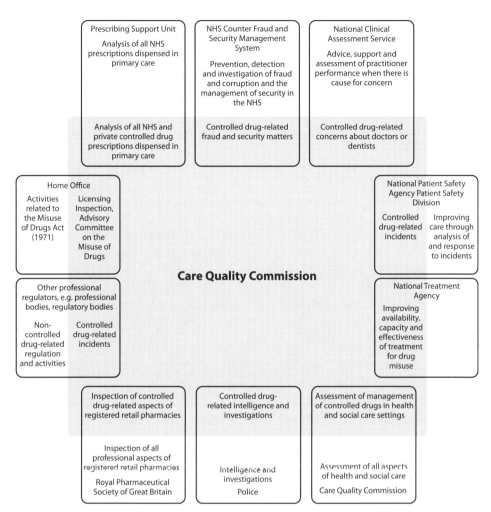

Figure 14.1 The agencies that are involved in different aspects of the regulation and control of controlled drugs. Reproduced with permission from the CQC, 2009.[34]

may be responsible for the deaths of 0.15% of all patients admitted to hospital.[35] Pharmacovigilance involves identifying a potential ADR that may be associated with a medicine, characterising it, evaluating the risks and benefits of the medicine, assessing the risks of taking action to change the availability of the medicine or information about it, then making a decision on action and communicating this to health professionals and the public. Most countries have some scheme in place and many send data from these schemes to a central monitoring centre in Sweden, the WHO Uppsala Monitoring Centre (WHO-UMC).

Yellow Card Scheme

The main pharmacovigilance system in the UK is the Yellow Card Scheme (YCS), run by the Medicines and Healthcare products Regulatory Agency (MHRA) to which pharmacists along with doctors, other health professionals and coroners, can submit reports of suspected ADRs identified in patients with whom they have had contact. The general public have also been able to report directly since 2005. It is not essential to be certain that there is an association between the medicine and the reaction to submit a report, only a suspicion. Information from Yellow Card reports is entered into a database ('Sentinel') and further information is sought from reporters if required to enable the report to be assessed. Reactions listed on the forms are categorised using the Medical Dictionary for Regulatory Affairs (MedDRA), a hierarchical method of grouping signs and symptoms, which is used internationally. The WHO also use a subset of adverse reaction terms (ARTs) for serious disease states, which have been regarded as particularly important to monitor, called WHO-ART.

Reports are assessed for causality, i.e. the likelihood that the problem was caused by the medicine, by expert staff at the MHRA. A variety of factors need to be considered in assessing causality.

- *Nature of the reaction:* some clinical events are commonly caused by medicines, such as Stevens Johnson syndrome.
- *Timing of the reaction:* some events occur minutes or hours after taking a single dose and are thus likely to be associated, although other events can be considerably delayed, even by years.
- *Relationship to dose:* if the dose changes, corresponding changes in the severity of the event may indicate an association.
- *Exclusion of other possible causes:* other medicines being taken or symptoms associated with disease states present should be considered as possible causes.

A systematic review has identified 34 different methods for assessing causality,[36] and studies have repeatedly shown that they lack consistency in the probabilities of particular drugs causing particular reactions. The categories used by the WHO-UMC are shown in Table 14.3.[37]

Signal generation, validation and strengthening

The reports are used to generate signals, i.e. the first alerts that there may be a problem with a medicine. A signal is defined by WHO-UMC as: 'reported information on a possible causal relationship between an adverse event and a drug, the relationship being unknown or incompletely documented previously. Usually more than a single report is required to generate a signal, depending upon the seriousness of the event and the quality of the

Table 14.3 World Health Organization categories of causality of suspected adverse drug reactions	
Causality category	**Assessment criteria**
Certain	Event or result with plausible time relationship to drug administration
	Cannot be explained by concurrent disease or other concomitant drugs
	When withdrawn (de-challenge) response is clinically plausible
	Event pharmacologically or phenomenologically definitive on re-challenge
Probable/likely	Event or result with a reasonable time relationship to drug administration
	Unlikely to be explained by concurrent disease or other concomitant drugs
	Follows a clinically reasonable response on withdrawal (dechallenge)
Possible	Event or result with a reasonable time relationship to drug administration
	Could also be explained by concurrent disease or other concomitant drugs
	Information on withdrawal (dechallenge) unclear or lacking
Unlikely	Event or result with a time relationship to drug administration which makes a relationship improbable, but not impossible
	Concurrent disease or other concomitant drugs provide plausible explanations
Conditional/unclassified	More data essential for classification
Unassessable/unclassifiable	Information insufficient or contradictory
	Data cannot be supplemented or verified
Adapted from reference 37.	

information.' Signals are more likely to be generated when events are reported for frequently used medicines, when the event described is normally rare and/ or often drug related, and when events occur in patients with similar characteristics. Many signals are generated automatically by the software each week, which depend on the number of reports submitted, which is constantly increasing. Different methods are used to generate signals, and it is possible for a signal to change as further reports are received. Obviously the length of time it takes for a signal to be generated will depend on the number of reports of the medicine and particular event received. This in turn depends on the frequency with which a medicines is used, as well as the number of people who actually submit reports. Hence the more people who submit reports, the greater the possibility of signals being detected earlier.

Staff regularly review the signals generated, to consider the extent of further work required. This may include requesting further details from reporters to enable causality assessment, contacting manufacturers to elicit any further information to support the association and reviewing the literature or other reporting databases.

Managing the findings

If a signal is confirmed as a potential ADR, then action may be required. This will vary depending on a number of factors including, the seriousness of the potential ADR, the likely incidence, which will be affected by the use of the medicine and the potential impact on health for the population, which will relate to the type of patient using the medicine. It is also important to consider whether other therapies are available to manage the condition(s) for which the medicine is being used and the risks associated with these conditions themselves. Possible actions which may result from identification of a new ADR are to amend the summary of product characteristics and/or the patient information leaflet for all products containing the drug in question, restricting usage or withdrawing marketing authorisation of the medicine.

Obviously if any of these actions are taken, it is essential to inform both health professionals and the public. The MHRA produces regular bulletins *Drug Safety Update* available on their website.[38] For individual issues, *Dear Doctor* letters are produced. These are published on the internet and also cascaded down through the Chief Medical Officer system, through NHS trusts and public health departments, to reach individual health professionals, including hospital staff, GPs and community pharmacists.

New products

Medicines newly introduced on to the UK market are given 'black triangle' status. These include entirely new drugs, new formulations of existing drugs or sometimes existing medicines that have new indications. All require intensive monitoring by the MHRA to further assess their risk/benefit profile and the time over which black triangle status is maintained varies, depending on how much information is obtained to ensure a product's continued safety. Many countries have similar systems for newly marketed products, which permit authorities to collect information about any problems with the product in their own country, even if the products have been marketed elsewhere.

Disadvantages of spontaneous reporting

The YCS, as with most spontaneous reporting systems, suffers from severe under-reporting, estimated by a systematic review as being 82–98%.[39]

Studies have shown a variety of reasons may be involved in under-reporting, including lack of certainty that the medicine caused the symptom, guilt feelings, fear of reprisal and apathy. Many possible methods of increasing reporting have been mooted over the years. One method, which includes ADR reporting as part of the overall quality of prescribing and rewards this with financial incentives, has recently been reported to result in higher than usual reporting rates.[14]

YCS data cannot provide the incidence of any individual ADR from any medicine, partly because of under-reporting, but also because the number of patients prescribed a particular drug is not known. Although data is freely available on the overall number of reports submitted in relation to a particular product, via drug analysis prints, from the MHRA website,[40] the data do not present a full analysis of risks and benefits associated with medicines. Hence health professionals, including pharmacists must be in a position to interpret the data for patients presenting with concerns about suspected ADRs.

Manufacturer responsibilities

MHRA also has a pharmacovigilance inspectorate, which assess the compliance of pharmaceutical manufacturers with legislation relating to the safety of medicines. This legislation is beyond the scope of this book. However, it should be noted that manufacturers are legally obliged to report any serious, unexpected ADR, from any clinical or epidemiological study, drug use or literature report within 15 days. Fatal or life-threatening ADRs must be reported within seven days. In addition, periodic safety update reports must be submitted every six months for the first two years after marketing, then with decreasing frequency to ensure the continued safety of marketed products.

Direct patient reporting

As already mentioned, MHRA accepts reports directly from patients and other members of the public. An evaluation of this has recently been completed which shows that there is limited awareness of the facility by both the public and among health professionals, but that most patient reporters learnt about the facility from pharmacies.[41] The majority of people who reported a suspected ADR identified it as such through issues relating to timing, as outlined in the causality methods used by pharmacovigilance experts, or by accessing information about the medicine, such as their patient information leaflet.[42] There is an increasing number of countries worldwide that accept patients reports. It has been suggested that there are advantages such as faster signal generation, avoiding the filtering effect of interpretation of events by health professionals and not least, maintaining the number of reports at a time when health professional reporting may be reducing.

Other reporting schemes

As outlined above, the WHO-UMC accepts reports from 96 countries, including the UK via the MHRA. Approximately 4.7 million reports are collated in the UMC database. In the USA, the Food and Drug Agency runs the MedWatch system, which, in addition to ADRs, also covers problems with products and medication errors. The MHRA operates the Defective Medicines Report Centre, which accepts reports concerning problems with medicines and also covers problems with medical devices, while, as outlined above, medication errors are reported to the NPSA in the UK. All alerts issued by the MHRA and the DoH, which includes messages from the Chief Medical Officer, and by NPSA are available on a single website, the Central Alerting System.[43] This site therefore has all details of safety alerts, drug recalls, *Dear Doctor* letters and medical device alerts issued.

Prescription event monitoring is a complementary pharmacovigilance system which is operated by the Drug Safety Research Unit at Southampton University.[44] This system involves the distribution of green forms to selected GP prescribers throughout the UK who have issued a prescription for a particular product. Products are selected specifically for monitoring, thus as a system it complements the YCS. GPs are asked to report on the green forms all events that have been reported to them by the patients prescribed the drug being studied since it was initiated over a specified time period, regardless of any suspected association of the event with the medicine. Since the number of patients is available as a denominator, prescription event monitoring has the ability to estimate the incidence of ADRs for these drugs and has been shown to identify new ADRs not previously suspected to be due to the drugs studied.

Pharmacist's role in pharmacovigilance

Pharmacists have many opportunities to identify suspected ADRs themselves and to support patients and other health professionals in doing so. Their role in explaining risks and benefits of medicines to patients (Chapter 10) is important in helping patients to understand the literature about and risks of ADRs. However, pharmacists should also routinely ask patients about problems with medicines including ADRs, and encourage patients to report or report themselves, since pharmacovigilance is a vital public health service.

Communicating medicines management issues

Ensuring the safe and effective use of medicines involves communicating with people, both patients and health professionals. Often this may be for the purpose of encouraging behaviour change. Some types of intervention designed to support behaviour change are described in Chapter 11. However, achieving change in prescribing behaviour may require other approaches. Involvement in the local development of formularies and treatment protocols encourages their use, but even where there is agreement in principle with these tools, there may still be resistance to change among both prescribers and patients.[5] Pharmacists are often actively involved in persuading prescribers to carry out changes and while the goal of rational, cost-effective prescribing may appeal to some, others may be swayed through such factors as peer pressure, the need to follow expert advice or of having influence themselves on others, personal achievement, financial gain or fear of litigation.

Patients are also increasingly aware of the drive to use cheaper alternative products for the same health gain, and pharmacists may be in a position to influence their behaviour, perhaps when prescriptions that have been changed for this purpose are presented for dispensing. Explaining the concepts of cost-effectiveness and maximising the use of scarce resources is therefore of importance to patients as well as to health professionals.

Understanding that there are many reasons for resistance to change and that people do differ in their drivers for change is important, since techniques needed to influence behaviour will need to vary as a result. Change itself is threatening and can take time. Changing prescribing behaviour, just like helping someone to stop smoking, may take repeated attempts and ensuring that prescribing is in line with local formularies and guidelines also requires constant intervention. An awareness of how to influence behaviour is obviously an asset for any pharmacist involved in public health. Chapter 10 highlights some ways in which pharmacists can help to bring about changes to practice, and there are many more suggestions on the National Institute for Health Research Service Delivery and Organisation website[45] and NICE guidance is also available on how to change practice.[46] However, over 150 systematic reviews have been conducted on behaviour change interventions. Many reviews of relevance are available on the Cochrane database. The message seems to be that there is no simple answer!

References

1. National Prescribing Centre. *Moving Towards Personalising Medicines Management: Improving outcomes for people through the safe and effective use of medicines.* Liverpool: NPC, 2008.
2. Garattini S, Bertele V, Godman B *et al.* Enhancing the rational use of new medicines across European healthcare systems: a position paper. *Eur J Clin Pharmacol* 2008; 64: 1137–1138.
3. World Health Organization (2010). *Rational Use of Medicines.* Geneva: WHO. http://www.who.int/medicines/areas/rational_use/en/index.html
4. Audit Commission. *Primary Care Prescribing: A bulletin for Primary Care Trusts.* London: Audit Commission, 2003.
5. Wettermark B, Godman B, Jacobsson B *et al.* Soft regulations in pharmaceutical policy making. *Appl Health Econ Health Pol* 2009; 7(3): 137–147.

6. Ostini R, Hegney D, Jackson C *et al*. Systematic review of interventions to improve prescribing. *Ann Pharmacother* 2008; 43: 502–513.

7. World Health Organization. *Model List of Essential Medicines*, 16th edn. Geneva: WHO, 2009. http://www.who.int/medicines/publications/essentialmedicines/en/index.html

8. Godman B, Bucsics Burkhardt T, Haycox A *et al*. Insight into recent reforms and initiatives in Austria: implications for key stakeholders. *Expert Rev Pharmacoeconom Outcomes Res* 2008; 8: 357–371.

9. Godman B, Wettermark B, Hoffman M *et al*. Multifaceted national and regional reforms in ambulatory care in Sweden: global relevance. *Expert Rev Pharmacoeconom Outcomes Res* 2009; 9: 65–83.

10. Sermet C, Andrieu V, Godman B *et al*. Ongoing pharmaceutical reforms in France: implications for key stakeholder groups. *Appl Health Econ Health Policy* 2010; 8: 7–24.

11. Anon. Do formularies work? *Bandolier* 2002; 9(4): 7.

12. Norman C, Zarrinkoub R, Hasselström J *et al*. Potential savings without compromising the quality of care. *Int J Clin Pract* 2009; 63: 1320–1326.

13. Krska J. In: Winfield A, Rees J, Smith I (eds). *Pharmaceutical Practice*, 4th ed. London: Churchill Livingstone, 2009.

14. Wettermark B, Pehrsson A, Juhasz-Haverinen M *et al*. Financial incentives linked to self-assessment of prescribing patterns: a new approach for quality improvement on drug prescribing in primary care. *Qual Primary Care* 2009; 17: 179–189.

15. Scottish Intercollegiate Guidelines Network. SIGN 50. *A Guideline Developer's Handbook* 2008. http://www.sign.ac.uk/guidelines/fulltext/50/index.html

16. Brouwers MC, Kho ME, Browman GP *et al*. Development of the AGREE II. *Can Med Assoc J*, 31 May 2010. doi: 10.1503/cmaj.091714.

17. Department of Health. *Quality and Outcomes Framework of the General Medical Services Contract*. London: DoH. http://www.dh.gov.uk/en/Healthcare/Primarycare/Primarycarecontracting/QOF/index.htm

18. National Institute for Health and Clinical Excellence (2010). *NICE Guideline Implementation Tools*. London: NICE. www.nice.org.uk/page.aspx?o=implementationadvice

19. National Institute for Health and Clinical Excellence (2010). *NICE Guideline Audit Tools*. London: NICE. www.nice.org.uk/page.aspx?o=auditcriteria

20. Zermansky AG. Who controls repeats? *Br J Gen Pract* 1996; 46: 643–637.

21. Halliday J *et al*. A framework for an ideal repeat prescribing system. *Pharm J* 2002; 268: 842–843.

22. Krska J, Gill D, Hansford D. Can pharmacists help GPs to do better medication reviews? A pharmacist supported medication review training package for GPs: an evaluation of documented issues and outputs and a postal questionnaire of GP views *Med Educ* 2006; 40: 1217–1225.

23. Hansford D, Krska J, Gill D *et al*. A training package for primary care nurses in conducting medication reviews: their views and the resultant outputs. *J Clin Nurs* 2008; 18: 1096–1104.

24. National Institute for Health and Clinical Excellence (2010). *Costing Tools*. London: NICE. www.nice.org.uk/page.aspx?o=costingtools

25. Department of Health (2007). *Strategies to Achieve Cost-Effective Prescribing: interim guidance for primary care trusts*. http://www.dh.gov.uk/en/Publicationsandstatistics/Publications/PublicationsPolicyAndGuidance/DH_076350

26. Department of Health (2006). *Good Practice Guidance on Managing the Introduction of New Healthcare Interventions and Links to NICE Technology Appraisal Guidance*. London: DoH. www.dh.gov.uk/en/Publicationsandstatistics/Publications/PublicationsPolicyAndGuidance/DH_064983

27. National Prescribing Centre. *Managing Medicines Across a Health Community: a fitness for purpose framework for area prescribing and medicines management committees*. Liverpool: NPC, 2009.

28. National Patient Safety Agency (2009). *Safer Lithium Therapy*. London: NPSA. http://www.nrls.npsa.nhs.uk/resources/type/alerts/?entryid45=65426

29. National Institute for Health and Clinical Excellence/National Patient Safety Agency (2007). *Technical Patient Safety Solutions for Medicines Reconciliation on Admission of Adults to Hospital: Guidance.* London: NICE/NPSA.
http://www.nice.org.uk/guidance/index.jsp?action=byID&o=11897

30. Care Quality Commission. *Managing Patients' Medicines After Discharge from Hospital.* London: QCC, 2009.

31. Craig J, Callen J, Marks A *et al.* Electronic discharge summaries: the current state of play. *HIM J* 2007; 36(3): 30–36.

32. National Health Service. *Connecting for Health. Summary Care Records.* London: NHS.
http://www.connectingforhealth.nhs.uk/systemsandservices/scr

33. Royal Pharmaceutical Society of Great Britain. *The Handling of Medicines in Social Care.* London: RPSGB, 2007.

34. Care Quality Commission. *The Safer Management of Controlled Drugs Annual Report.* London: QCC, 2008.

35. Pirmohamed M *et al.* Adverse drug reactions as cause of admission to hospital: prospective analysis of 18 820 patients. *BMJ* 2004; 329: 15–19.

36. Agbabiaki TB, Savovic J, Ernst E. Methods for causality assessment of adverse drug reactions. *Drug Safety* 2008; 31: 21–37.

37. World Health Organization Uppsala Monitoring Centre. Causality Categories. Uppsala: WHO-UMC. http://www.who-umc.org/DynPage.aspx?id=22682

38. Medicines and Healthcare Products Regulatory Agency and Commission on Human Medicines. *Drug Safety Update.* London: MRHA.
http://www.mhra.gov.uk/Publications/Safetyguidance/DrugSafetyUpdate/index.htm

39. Hazell L, Shakir SAW. Under-reporting of adverse drug reactions: a systematic review. *Drug Safety* 2006; 29(5): 385–396.

40. Medicines and Healthcare Products Regulatory Agency. *Drug Analysis.* London: MRHA.
http://www.mhra.gov.uk/Onlineservices/Medicines/Druganalysisprints/index.htm

41. McLernon D, Lee AJ, Watson MC *et al.* Consumer reporters' views and attitudes towards the Yellow Card Scheme for Adverse Drug Reaction reports: a questionnaire study. *Int J Pharm Pract* 2009; 17(Suppl2): B25–26.

42. Krska J, Taylor J, Avery AJ. How do patients identify ADRs? A quantitative analysis in reporters to the Yellow Card Scheme. *Pharmacoepi Drug Saf* 2010; 19 652.

43. National Health Service. *Central Alerting System.* London: NHS. https://www.cas.dh.gov.uk/Home.aspx

44. Drug Safety Research Unit. Prescription-Event Monitoring (PEM). Southampton: DSRU.
http://www.dsru.org/pem/prescriptioneventmonitoringpem.html?
PHPSESSID=4eb1c7591adea8ab8b874ba783ad3c88

45. National Institute for Health Research Service Delivery and Organisation Programme. *Managing Change in the NHS.* Southampton: NIHR.
http://www.sdo.nihr.ac.uk/managingchange.html

46. National Institute for Health and Clinical Excellence. *How to Change Practice: understand, identify and overcome barriers to change.* London: NICE, 2009.

Glossary

Acronym	Full name	Definition
ARR	absolute risk reduction	arithmetic difference in outcome rates for two groups in a clinical trial
BMI	body mass index	calculated as mass (kg) divided by height squared (m)
CEA	cost-effectiveness analysis	economic evaluation of two interventions with differing benefits measured in the same units
CMA	cost-minimisation analysis	economic evaluation of two interventions with the same benefits
CUA	cost-utility analysis	a form of CEA in which the consequences are measured in terms of quality-adjusted life-years
DALY	disability-adjusted life-year	a year of healthy life lost through either early death or disability
DDD	defined daily dose	the average recommended daily maintenance dose for a drug when used for its most common indication in adults
ICER	incremental cost-effectiveness ratio	difference between the costs of two interventions divided by the difference between the benefits of these two interventions
IMD	index of multiple deprivation	a combined indicator which covers economic, social and housing issues, available for output areas throughout England

NNH	number needed to harm	the number of patients that need to be treated for one to be harmed, compared with a control
NNT	number need to treat	the number of patients that need to be treated for one to benefit, compared with a control; calculated as the reciprocal of the ARR
OA	output area	geographical areas defined by the 2001 Census for which information about IMD is available
OR	odds ratio	the ratio of the odds of having a particular outcome in two study groups: intervention and control
PPV	positive predictive value	proportion of people who are tested for a condition who actually have the condition
PYLL	potential years life lost	an estimate of the years lost through early death
QALY	quality-adjusted life-year	a measure which incorporates both the quality and quantity of life
RR	relative risk	the ratio of risk in a treated group compared to a control group in a clinical study
RRR	relative risk reduction	the difference between risks in two groups in a study divided by the risk in the control group

Index